Arthritis Cookbooks recipe

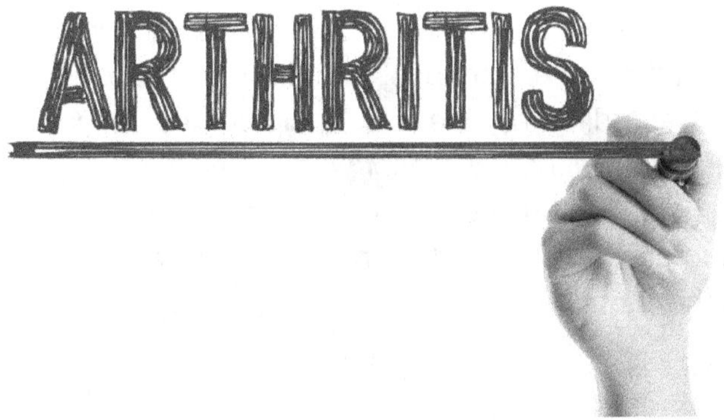

Ultimate Delicious Recipes for Joint Health and Pain Relief

Violet M. Schulze

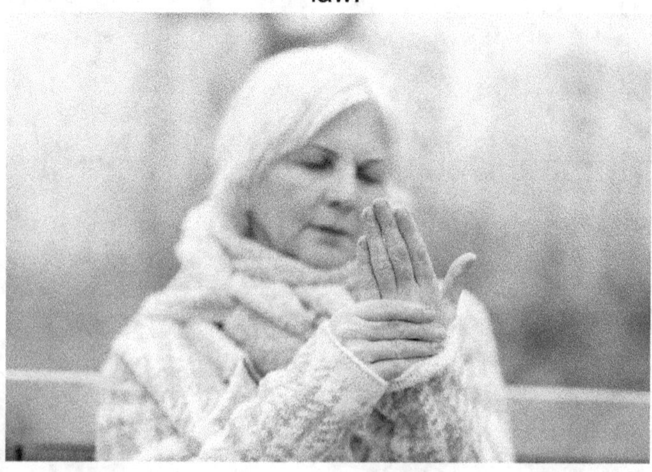

Table of contents

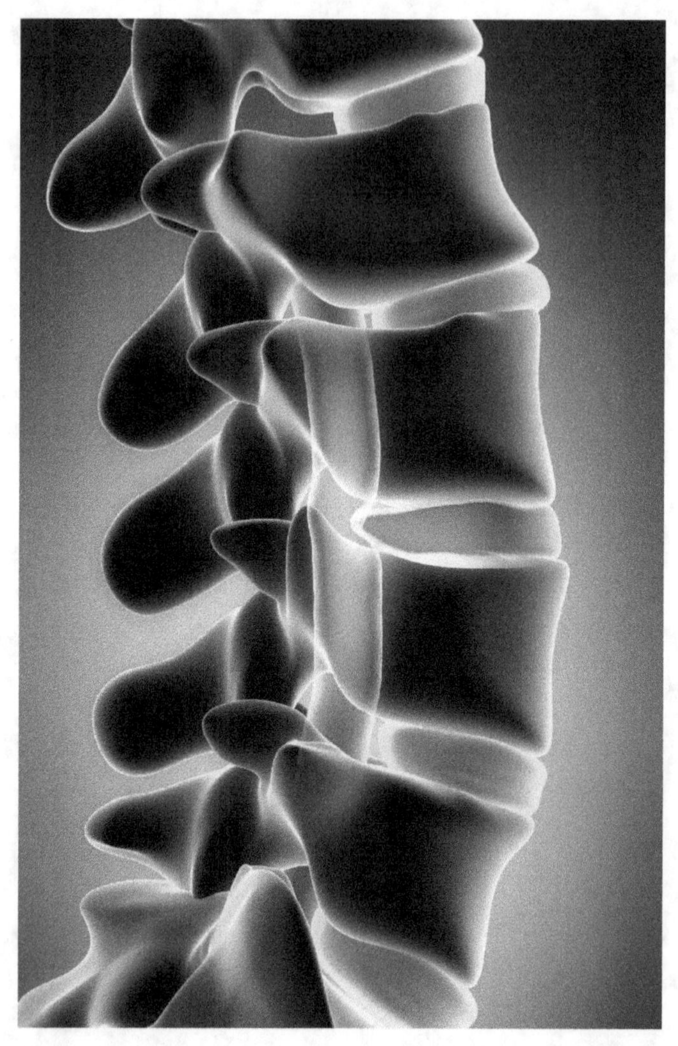

INTRODUCTIO

N

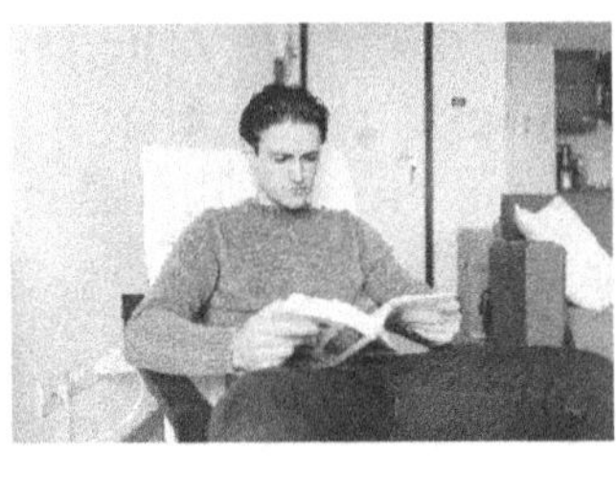 A sigh escaped John's lips as he sat in his favorite armchair, a book on his lap. His arthritis had recently worsened, producing joint discomfort and stiffness. Simple things like holding a spoon or clutching a knife have become difficult. John had always enjoyed cooking, but his illness made it impossible for him to do so.

He came upon a recommendation for an arthritis recipe while scrolling through an online forum for arthritis sufferers. He followed the link, which led him to a website dedicated to assisting people with arthritis improve their quality of life via nutrition.

The cookbook included dishes to reduce inflammation, relieve joint pain, and promote general joint health. John decided it was worth a risk and ordered a copy, eagerly awaiting its arrival. He couldn't wait to get his hands on the book and learn the secrets it held.

John's first recipe was a robust vegetable soup. He sliced the veggies into small, manageable pieces with the help of the cookbook, easing pressure on his hands. He followed the recipe's instructions, including anti-inflammatory herbs and spices. He felt a spark of excitement that he hadn't felt in a long time as the aroma filled his kitchen.

He was astounded when he took his first spoonful. He could feel the warmth and food soaking into his bones as the flavors swirled on his tongue. The pain that usually accompanied each movement vanished, replaced by a calming sensation. It was as if the cookbook had cast a spell on him, bestowing relief and delight.

Encouraged by his initial success, John began to experiment with the recipes in the booklet. He discovered delectable foods like grilled salmon with turmeric, quinoa salad with avocado and kale, and even anti-inflammatory treats like berries and dark chocolate. Each recipe was meticulously created to be both healthful and delicious to the taste senses.

John quickly found himself spending an increasing amount of time in the kitchen. He experimented with ingredients, tailoring recipes to his specific preferences and nutritional requirements. He shared his newfound interest with colleagues and family by holding small gatherings and serving foods from the arthritis cookbook. Their compliments and smiles inspired his drive to overcome his illness.

As the months passed, John's arthritis symptoms improved significantly. The discomfort became more bearable, and he regained some of his lost mobility. He ascribed these beneficial developments to the cookbook's therapeutic ability. Inspired by his own transformation, he began a blog to share his experience with those suffering from arthritis.

John's blog quickly gained popularity, and he soon had a devoted following of readers looking for advice and inspiration. Many of them bought the arthritis cookbook and began their own cooking journeys. John's tale became a beacon of hope, demonstrating that it was possible to regain one's life from the clutches of arthritis with the correct information and drive.

As John sat back in his armchair, this time with his laptop open to his blog, he couldn't help but think about how far he'd come. The arthritis cookbook not only transformed his relationship with food, but it also sparked a desire to help others. He had become a source of inspiration and encouragement for numerous folks on their own arthritis journeys by sharing his stories and the healing power of the cookbook.

At that time, John was overwhelmed with appreciation for the arthritis cookbook and the fellowship it had brought into his life. He vowed to continue his mission of sharing optimism and showing others that arthritis did not have to define their lives with newfound vigor and purpose.

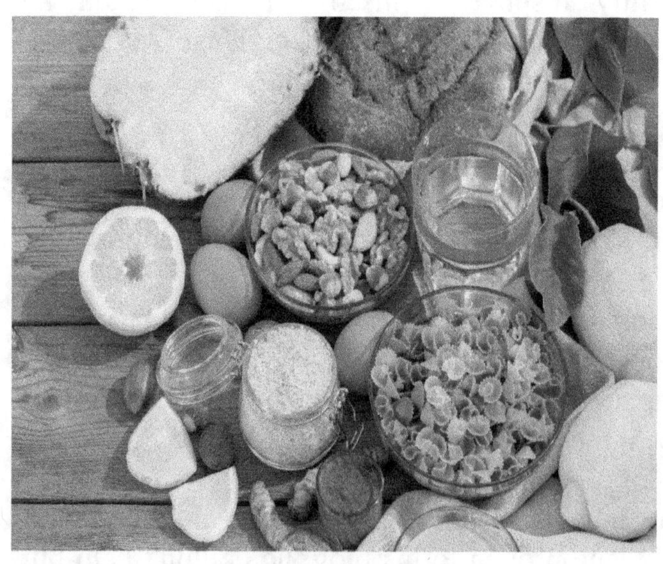

CHAPTER 1: BREAKFAST AND BRUNCH RECIPES

Oatmeal with Berries

Ingredients:

- 1 cup rolled oats
- 2 cups water
- Pinch of salt
- 1 cup mixed berries (such as strawberries, blueberries, raspberries)
- 2 tablespoons honey or maple syrup (optional)
- 1 tablespoon chia seeds (optional)
- 1/4 cup chopped nuts (such as almonds, walnuts, or pecans) (optional)
- Milk or yogurt for serving (optional)

Instructions:

1. In a saucepan, bring the water to a boil. Add a pinch of salt.
2. Stir in the rolled oats and reduce the heat to low. Simmer for about 5 minutes, stirring occasionally, until the oats are cooked and have absorbed most of the water. Adjust the cooking time according

to the instructions on the oatmeal package, if needed.

3. While the oats are cooking, wash the berries and chop any larger fruits into bite-sized pieces.
4. Once the oatmeal is cooked, remove the saucepan from the heat. If desired, stir in honey or maple syrup to sweeten the oatmeal.
5. To assemble, divide the cooked oatmeal into serving bowls. Top each bowl with a handful of mixed berries and sprinkle with chia seeds and chopped nuts, if using.
6. Serve the oatmeal with berries warm. If desired, drizzle some milk or yogurt over the top for added creaminess.

Greek Yogurt Parfait

Ingredients:

- 1 cup Greek yogurt
- 1 tablespoon honey or maple syrup
- 1/2 teaspoon vanilla extract
- 1 cup granola
- 1 cup mixed berries (strawberries, blueberries, raspberries)
- Fresh mint leaves (optional, for garnish)

Instructions:

1. In a mixing dish, add the Greek yogurt, honey (or maple syrup), and vanilla extract. This will serve as the foundation for your parfait.
2. Begin layering the ingredients in a glass or clear container. Begin by layering a dollop of the Greek yogurt mixture on the bottom.
3. Sprinkle granola on top of the yogurt. You can use your favorite granola or make your own from scratch.
4. Then, top with a layer of mixed berries. You can use either fresh or frozen berries, depending on your preference. Slice larger berries, such as strawberries, into smaller pieces.
5. Layer the granola and berries on top of another tablespoon of the Greek yogurt mixture. Continue layering until the top of the glass or container is reached.
6. Finish with a final dollop of Greek yogurt on top and, if wanted, sprinkle with a few fresh mint leaves.
7. Enjoy the refreshing and tasty Greek Yogurt Parfait right away!

Vegetable Omelet

Ingredients:

- 3 eggs
- 1/4 cup diced onion
- 1/4 cup diced bell pepper (any color)
- 1/4 cup diced tomato
- 1/4 cup sliced mushrooms
- 1/4 cup chopped spinach
- Salt and pepper to taste
- 1 tablespoon butter or cooking oil
- Optional: shredded cheese (such as cheddar or feta) for topping

Instructions:

1. Melt the butter or frying oil in a nonstick skillet over medium heat, allowing it to cover the pan evenly.
2. In a mixing basin, thoroughly combine the eggs. Season with salt and pepper to your liking.
3. To the skillet, add the diced onion, bell pepper, tomato, mushrooms, and spinach. Cook for 5 minutes, or until the vegetables are soft.
4. Turn off the heat and pour the beaten eggs over the sautéed vegetables. Allow the eggs to cook evenly in the skillet.

5. Cook for 2-3 minutes, or until the edges begin to set. Lift the edges of the skillet gently with a spatula and tilt the skillet to allow the raw eggs to flow to the edges.
6. When the omelet is mostly set but still little runny on top, add the optional shredded cheese to one side.
7. Fold the omelet in half carefully with the spatula, covering the side with the cheese (if using). Gently press down.
8. Cook for 1 minute more, or until the cheese melts and the omelet is done.
9. Place the omelet on a platter to serve. If desired, top with more chopped vegetables or herbs.
10. As a healthy breakfast or brunch alternative, serve the vegetable omelet warm. It goes nicely with whole grain toast, a salad on the side, or fresh fruit.

Smoothie with Turmeric

Ingredients:

- 3 eggs
- 1/4 cup diced onion
- 1/4 cup diced bell pepper (any color)
- 1/4 cup diced tomato
- 1/4 cup sliced mushrooms
- 1/4 cup chopped spinach

- Salt and pepper to taste
- 1 tablespoon butter or cooking oil
- Optional: shredded cheese (such as cheddar or feta) for topping

Instructions:

1. Melt the butter or frying oil in a nonstick skillet over medium heat, allowing it to cover the pan evenly.
2. In a mixing basin, thoroughly combine the eggs. Season with salt and pepper to your liking.
3. To the skillet, add the diced onion, bell pepper, tomato, mushrooms, and spinach. Cook for 5 minutes, or until the vegetables are soft.
4. Turn off the heat and pour the beaten eggs over the sautéed vegetables. Allow the eggs to cook evenly in the skillet.
5. Cook for 2-3 minutes, or until the edges begin to set. Lift the edges of the skillet gently with a spatula and tilt the skillet to allow the raw eggs to flow to the edges.
6. When the omelet is mostly set but still little runny on top, add the optional shredded cheese to one side.
7. Fold the omelet in half carefully with the spatula, covering the side with the cheese (if using). Gently press down.

8. Cook for 1 minute more, or until the cheese melts and the omelet is done.
9. Place the omelet on a platter to serve. If desired, top with more chopped vegetables or herbs.
10. As a healthy breakfast or brunch alternative, serve the vegetable omelet warm. It goes nicely with whole grain toast, a salad on the side, or fresh fruit.

Avocado Toast

Ingredients:

- 2 slices of bread (whole grain or sourdough)
- 1 ripe avocado
- 1 tablespoon lemon juice
- Salt and pepper to taste
- Optional toppings: sliced cherry tomatoes, crumbled feta cheese, red pepper flakes, microgreens, etc.

Instructions:

1. Toast the bread slices to your preferred crispiness.

2. Cut the avocado in half, remove the pit, and spoon the flesh into a bowl as the bread toasts.
3. Mash the avocado with a fork until it reaches the consistency you like. You can leave it slightly lumpy or smooth it out.
4. Mix in the lemon juice with the mashed avocado. The lemon juice adds taste while also preventing browning of the avocado.
5. Season the avocado mixture to taste with salt and pepper. Seasoning can be adjusted to your liking.
6. After toasting the bread pieces, evenly sprinkle the mashed avocado on top of each slice.
7. It's now time to get creative with the garnishes! You can add sliced cherry tomatoes, crumbled feta cheese, or a dash of red pepper flakes for a spicy kick. Experiment with other toppings such as microgreens, sliced radishes, or even a fried egg.
8. Serve the avocado toast as soon as the bread is warm and crispy.

Quinoa Breakfast Bowl

Ingredients:

- 1 cup cooked quinoa
- 1 cup almond milk (or any milk of your choice)
- 1 tablespoon honey or maple syrup
- 1 teaspoon vanilla extract
- 1/2 teaspoon cinnamon
- 1 ripe banana, sliced
- 1/2 cup fresh berries (such as blueberries, strawberries, or raspberries)
- 2 tablespoons chopped nuts (such as almonds, walnuts, or pecans)
- 1 tablespoon chia seeds
- Optional toppings: shredded coconut, cocoa nibs, or additional honey/maple syrup

Instructions:

1. Combine the cooked quinoa, almond milk, honey or maple syrup, vanilla essence, and cinnamon in a small saucepan. To blend, stir everything together thoroughly.
2. Bring the mixture to a slow simmer in a saucepan over medium heat. Cook for 5 minutes, or until the quinoa has absorbed part of the liquid and has turned creamy. To avoid sticking, stir occasionally.

3. When the quinoa mixture has reached the required consistency, take it from the fire and set aside to cool somewhat.
4. Serve the quinoa mixture in individual bowls. Each bowl should be topped with sliced banana, fresh berries, chopped almonds, and chia seeds.
5. To enhance flavor and texture, sprinkle shredded coconut or cocoa nibs over top.
6. If desired, drizzle with more honey or maple syrup.
7. Enjoy your Quinoa Breakfast Bowls right away!

Chia Seed Pudding

Ingredients:

- 1/4 cup chia seeds
- 1 cup milk (dairy or plant-based)
- 2 tablespoons sweetener of your choice (honey, maple syrup, or agave nectar)
- 1/2 teaspoon vanilla extract
- Optional toppings: fresh fruits, nuts, shredded coconut, or granola

Instructions:

1. Combine the chia seeds, milk, sweetener, and vanilla extract in a medium-sized mixing dish.
2. To uniformly distribute the chia seeds, thoroughly whisk the mixture. Make certain that there are no clumps.
3. Allow the mixture to sit for 5 minutes before whisking again to prevent clumping.
4. Refrigerate the bowl for at least 2 hours or overnight. The chia seeds will absorb the liquid and thicken to form a pudding-like consistency during this period.
5. Give the pudding a thorough stir once it has set to break up any clumps that may have formed. If the consistency is too thick for you, thin it out with a little more milk.
6. Chia seed pudding should be served in individual bowls or glasses. To enhance flavor and texture, top with your favorite fruits, nuts, shredded coconut, or granola.
7. Enjoy your homemade chia seed pudding right away or save it in the refrigerator for later. It can be stored in the refrigerator for up to 3-4 days.

Ingredients:

- For the pancakes:

- 1 cup whole wheat flour
- 1/2 cup all-purpose flour
- 2 tablespoons sugar
- 2 teaspoons baking powder
- 1/2 teaspoon baking soda
- 1/2 teaspoon salt
- 1 cup buttermilk
- 1/2 cup milk
- 2 large eggs
- 2 tablespoons unsalted butter, melted
- 1 teaspoon vanilla extract

For the fruit compote:

- 2 cups mixed fresh berries (such as strawberries, blueberries, raspberries)
- 2 tablespoons sugar
- 2 tablespoons water
- 1 tablespoon lemon juice

Instructions:

1. Whisk together the whole wheat flour, all-purpose flour, sugar, baking powder,

baking soda, and salt in a large mixing basin.

2. Combine the buttermilk, milk, eggs, melted butter, and vanilla essence in a separate basin. Whisk until well combined.

3. Stir the wet components into the dry ingredients until they are barely mixed. It's fine if the batter has a few lumps.

4. Melt butter in a nonstick skillet or griddle over medium heat. Cooking spray or a little amount of butter should be used to lightly oil the surface.

5. For each pancake, pour 1/4 cup batter into the skillet. Cook until surface bubbles appear, then flip and cook for another 1-2 minutes, or until golden brown. Repeat with the rest of the batter.

6. Prepare the fruit compote while the pancakes are cooking. Combine the mixed berries, sugar, water, and lemon juice in a saucepan. Cook for about 5 minutes, or until the berries soften and release their juices, over medium heat. Stir every now and again.

7. Remove the fruit compote from the heat and set aside to cool. As it cools, the compote will thicken.

8. Serve with a big scoop of fruit compote on top of the whole-grain pancakes. If

desired, top with additional fresh fruit or drizzle with maple syrup.

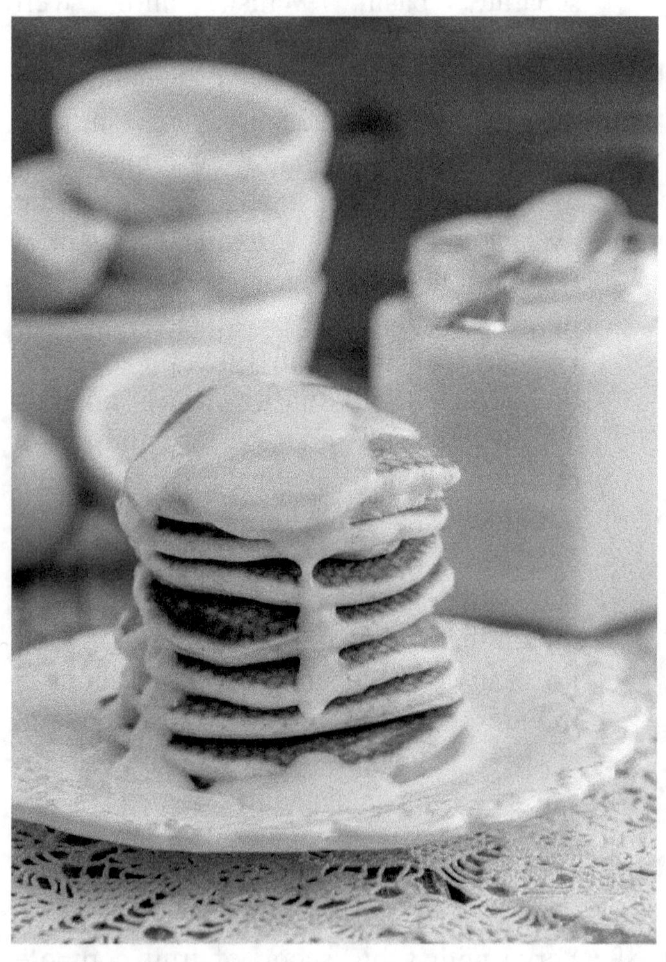

CHAPTER 2 : LUNCH RECIPES

Quinoa Salad

Ingredients:

- 1 cup quinoa
- 2 cups water
- 1 cucumber, diced
- 1 red bell pepper, diced
- 1 yellow bell pepper, diced
- 1 small red onion, finely chopped
- 1 cup cherry tomatoes, halved
- 1/2 cup fresh parsley, chopped
- 1/4 cup fresh mint leaves, chopped
- 1/4 cup feta cheese, crumbled
- 1/4 cup kalamata olives, pitted and sliced (optional)
- 1/4 cup extra-virgin olive oil
- 2 tablespoons lemon juice
- 2 cloves garlic, minced
- Salt and pepper to taste

Instructions:

1. To remove any bitterness from the quinoa, thoroughly rinse it under cold

water. Bring the water to a boil in a saucepan and add the quinoa. Reduce the heat to low, cover, and leave to simmer for 15 minutes, or until all of the water has been absorbed. Remove from the heat and set aside to cool.

2. Combine the cooked quinoa, diced cucumber, diced red and yellow bell peppers, chopped red onion, cherry tomatoes, parsley, and mint leaves in a large mixing dish.
3. To create the dressing, mix together the olive oil, lemon juice, minced garlic, salt, and pepper in a small bowl.
4. Pour the dressing over the quinoa mixture and gently toss to coat all of the ingredients.
5. Gently combine the salad with the crumbled feta cheese and kalamata olives (if using).
6. Season with salt and pepper to taste.
7. Refrigerate the bowl, covered with plastic wrap, for at least 30 minutes to enable the flavors to mingle.
8. Chill and serve as a pleasant and nutritious salad.

Salmon Wrap

Ingredients:

- 2 large tortilla wraps
- 2 salmon fillets
- 1 tablespoon olive oil
- Salt and pepper to taste
- 1/2 cup Greek yogurt
- 2 tablespoons lemon juice
- 1 tablespoon chopped dill
- 1 cup shredded lettuce
- 1/2 cup sliced cucumbers
- 1/2 cup sliced tomatoes
- 1/4 cup sliced red onions
- 1/4 cup sliced avocado

Instructions:

1. Preheat the oven to 400 degrees Fahrenheit (200 degrees Celsius). Line a baking sheet with parchment paper and place the salmon fillets on it. Drizzle olive oil over the fillets and season to taste with salt and pepper.
2. Bake the salmon for 12-15 minutes, or until cooked through and flaky, in a preheated oven. Remove from the oven and set aside to cool.
3. Combine the Greek yogurt, lemon juice, and dill in a small bowl. To make the sauce, combine all of the ingredients in a mixing bowl.
4. Spread a liberal amount of Greek yogurt sauce over one tortilla wrap.

5. In the center of the tortilla wrap, arrange half of the shredded lettuce, cucumber slices, tomatoes, red onions, and avocado in a row.
6. Place half of the cooked salmon on top of the vegetables, flaked into bite-sized pieces.
7. Fold the tortilla wrap's sides over the filling, then roll it up tightly from one end to the other to form a wrap.
8. Steps 4–7 should be repeated with the remaining tortilla wrap and ingredients.
9. If desired, cut each wrap in half diagonally and serve immediately.

Vegetable Stir-Fry

Ingredients:

- 2 tablespoons vegetable oil
- 1 onion, thinly sliced
- 2 cloves of garlic, minced
- 1 bell pepper, thinly sliced
- 2 carrots, julienned
- 1 zucchini, sliced
- 1 cup broccoli florets
- 1 cup snap peas

- 1 cup mushrooms, sliced
- 1 cup baby corn, halved
- 1/4 cup soy sauce
- 2 tablespoons oyster sauce (optional)
- 1 tablespoon cornstarch, dissolved in 2 tablespoons water
- Salt and pepper to taste
- Sesame seeds for garnish (optional)

Instructions:

1. In a large pan or wok, heat the vegetable oil over medium-high heat.
2. To the pan, add the sliced onion and minced garlic. Cook for 1-2 minutes, or until the onion is transparent.
3. To the pan, add the bell pepper, carrots, zucchini, broccoli, snap peas, mushrooms, and baby corn. Cook for 5-7 minutes, or until the vegetables are crisp-tender. You can modify the cooking time dependent on how soft you like your vegetables.
4. Combine the soy sauce and oyster sauce in a small bowl. Pour the sauce mixture into the pan with the vegetables. Stir to evenly coat the vegetables.
5. In a separate small bowl, make a slurry of cornstarch and water. Pour the slurry into the pan and give it a good swirl. This will aid in the thickening of the sauce.

6. Cook for a further 1-2 minutes, or until the sauce thickens and coats the vegetables. Season the stir-fry with salt and pepper to taste.
7. Remove the vegetable stir-fry from the pan and place it in a serving dish.
8. If desired, garnish with sesame seeds for extra taste and presentation.
9. Serve the vegetable stir-fry as a main course or as a side dish alongside steaming rice or noodles.

Lentil Soup

Ingredients:

- 1 cup dried lentils (green or brown)
- 1 onion, chopped
- 2 carrots, diced
- 2 celery stalks, diced
- 3 garlic cloves, minced
- 1 can diced tomatoes (14 oz)
- 4 cups vegetable broth
- 1 teaspoon ground cumin
- 1 teaspoon ground coriander
- 1/2 teaspoon turmeric
- 1/2 teaspoon paprika
- 1 bay leaf
- 2 tablespoons olive oil
- Salt and pepper to taste

- Fresh parsley or cilantro for garnish (optional)

Instructions:

1. Set aside the lentils after rinsing them in cold water.
2. In a large pot, heat the olive oil over medium heat. Combine the onion, carrots, celery, and garlic in a mixing bowl. Sauté the vegetables for 5-7 minutes, or until tender.
3. To the pot, add the cumin, coriander, turmeric, and paprika. Stir the spices into the vegetables thoroughly.
4. To the pot, add the lentils, diced tomatoes (including juice), vegetable broth, and bay leaf. Season to taste with salt and pepper.
5. Bring the soup to a boil, then lower to a low heat. Cover and cook for 30-40 minutes, or until the lentils are cooked.
6. Take the bay leaf out of the pot. If necessary, taste the soup and adjust the seasoning.
7. If you prefer a thicker soup, you can partially blend it with an immersion blender or extract about 1 cup of the broth and blend it in a conventional blender before returning it to the saucepan.

8. Serve the lentil soup hot, garnished if preferred with fresh parsley or cilantro.

Spinach and Mushroom Omelette

Ingredients:

- 3 large eggs
- 1 cup fresh spinach leaves, chopped
- 1/2 cup mushrooms, sliced
- 1/4 cup grated cheese (such as cheddar or Swiss)
- 1/4 cup milk
- 1 tablespoon butter or cooking oil
- Salt and pepper to taste

Instructions:

1. Melt the butter or cooking oil in a nonstick skillet over medium heat. Allow it to melt and uniformly coat the bottom of the skillet.
2. Whisk the eggs and milk together in a mixing basin until well mixed. Season with salt and pepper to your liking.
3. To the skillet, add the chopped spinach and sliced mushrooms. Sauté for 3-4 minutes, or until tender and any excess moisture has evaporated.

4. Pour the egg mixture over the skillet's sautéed spinach and mushrooms. Allow it to cook for about a minute, or until the edges begin to firm.
5. Lift the edges of the omelette lightly with a spatula and tilt the skillet to allow the uncooked egg mixture to flow to the edges. Cook for another 2-3 minutes, or until the omelette is mostly set but slightly runny on top.
6. Evenly distribute the grated cheese over one side of the omelette.
7. Fold the omelette in half carefully, covering one side with the cheese. Gently press down with the spatula to help the cheese melt.
8. Cook for an additional 1-2 minutes, or until the cheese is melted and the omelette is done to your liking.
9. Place the omelette on a plate and serve immediately. If desired, garnish with more chopped spinach or mushrooms.

Grilled Chicken Salad

Ingredients:

- 2 boneless, skinless chicken breasts
- 6 cups mixed salad greens (such as romaine lettuce, spinach, or arugula)

- 1 cup cherry tomatoes, halved
- 1/2 cup cucumber, sliced
- 1/4 cup red onion, thinly sliced
- 1/4 cup sliced black olives
- 1/4 cup crumbled feta cheese
- 2 tablespoons fresh lemon juice
- 2 tablespoons olive oil
- 1 clove garlic, minced
- 1 teaspoon dried oregano
- Salt and pepper to taste

Instructions:

1. Preheat the grill to medium-high.
2. Salt, pepper, and dried oregano season the chicken breasts. Drizzle with 1 tablespoon olive oil and rub the seasoning combination evenly over the chicken.
3. Grill the seasoned chicken breasts for 6-8 minutes per side, or until the chicken is cooked through and has reached an internal temperature of 165°F (74°C). Remove the chicken from the grill and set aside for a few minutes to rest.
4. Prepare the salad while the chicken is resting. Combine the salad greens, cherry tomatoes, cucumber, red onion, sliced black olives, and crumbled feta cheese in a large mixing basin.
5. To prepare the dressing, mix together the lemon juice, minced garlic, remaining

tablespoon olive oil, salt, and pepper in a small bowl.

6. Thinly slice the grilled chicken breasts.
7. Drizzle the dressing over the top of the salad with the cut chicken. Gently toss all of the ingredients in the dressing to coat.
8. Serve the salad on individual plates or bowls.
9. Enjoy the Grilled Chicken Salad immediately!

Chickpea and Vegetable Curry

Ingredients:

- 2 tablespoons vegetable oil
- 1 onion, diced
- 3 cloves of garlic, minced
- 1 tablespoon ginger, grated
- 1 red bell pepper, diced
- 1 zucchini, diced
- 1 cup cauliflower florets
- 1 cup broccoli florets
- 1 can (15 ounces) chickpeas, drained and rinsed
- 1 can (14 ounces) diced tomatoes
- 1 can (13.5 ounces) coconut milk
- 2 tablespoons curry powder
- 1 teaspoon turmeric powder
- 1 teaspoon cumin powder

- 1/2 teaspoon coriander powder
- 1/4 teaspoon cayenne pepper (optional, for heat)
- Salt and pepper to taste
- Fresh cilantro, chopped (for garnish)
- Cooked rice or naan bread (for serving)

Instructions:

1. In a large skillet or saucepan, heat the vegetable oil over medium heat.
2. Sauté the diced onion until it is transparent and slightly browned.
3. Cook for another minute, or until the minced garlic and grated ginger are aromatic.
4. To the skillet, add the diced red bell pepper, zucchini, cauliflower florets, and broccoli florets. Cook for about 5 minutes, or until the vegetables soften.
5. To the skillet, add the chickpeas, diced tomatoes (with juices), and coconut milk. To blend, stir everything together thoroughly.
6. Combine the curry powder, turmeric powder, cumin powder, coriander powder, cayenne pepper (if using), salt, and pepper in a small bowl. Stir the spice mixture into the skillet to coat the vegetables and chickpeas evenly.

7. Reduce the heat to low, cover the skillet, and cook for 15-20 minutes, or until the vegetables are soft.
8. Taste the curry and adjust the seasoning as needed, adding more salt, pepper, or spices to taste.
9. Remove the curry from the heat when it is done. Serve the chickpea and vegetable curry with naan bread or boiled rice.
10. To add freshness and taste, garnish with freshly chopped cilantro.

Turkey Lettuce Wraps

Ingredients:

- 2 tablespoons vegetable oil
- 1 onion, diced
- 3 cloves of garlic, minced
- 1 tablespoon ginger, grated
- 1 red bell pepper, diced
- 1 zucchini, diced
- 1 cup cauliflower florets
- 1 cup broccoli florets
- 1 can (15 ounces) chickpeas, drained and rinsed
- 1 can (14 ounces) diced tomatoes
- 1 can (13.5 ounces) coconut milk
- 2 tablespoons curry powder
- 1 teaspoon turmeric powder

- 1 teaspoon cumin powder
- 1/2 teaspoon coriander powder
- 1/4 teaspoon cayenne pepper (optional, for heat)
- Salt and pepper to taste
- Fresh cilantro, chopped (for garnish)
- Cooked rice or naan bread (for serving)

Instructions:

1. In a large skillet or saucepan, heat the vegetable oil over medium heat.
2. Sauté the diced onion until it is transparent and slightly browned.
3. Cook for another minute, or until the minced garlic and grated ginger are aromatic.
4. To the skillet, add the diced red bell pepper, zucchini, cauliflower florets, and broccoli florets. Cook for about 5 minutes, or until the vegetables soften.
5. To the skillet, add the chickpeas, diced tomatoes (with juices), and coconut milk. To blend, stir everything together thoroughly.
6. Combine the curry powder, turmeric powder, cumin powder, coriander powder, cayenne pepper (if using), salt, and pepper in a small bowl. Stir the spice mixture into the skillet to coat the vegetables and chickpeas evenly.

7. Reduce the heat to low, cover the skillet, and cook for 15-20 minutes, or until the vegetables are soft.
8. Taste the curry and adjust the seasoning as needed, adding more salt, pepper, or spices to taste.
9. Remove the curry from the heat when it is done. Serve the chickpea and vegetable curry with naan bread or boiled rice.
10. To add freshness and taste, garnish with freshly chopped cilantro.

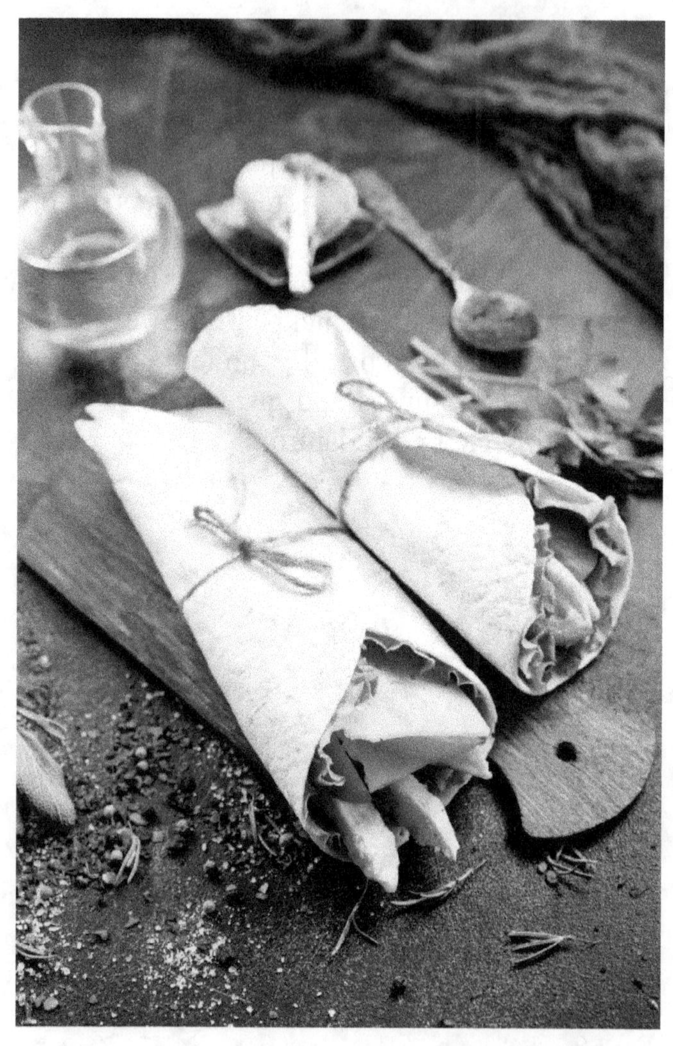

CHAPTER 3:DINNER RECIPES

Grilled Salmon with Quinoa Salad

Ingredients:

- 4 salmon fillets
- 1 cup quinoa
- 2 cups water or vegetable broth
- 1 cucumber, diced
- 1 red bell pepper, diced
- 1/2 red onion, finely chopped
- 1/4 cup fresh parsley, chopped
- 1/4 cup fresh mint leaves, chopped
- Juice of 1 lemon
- 2 tablespoons extra-virgin olive oil
- Salt and pepper to taste

Instructions:

1. Preheat the grill to medium-high.
2. To remove any bitterness from the quinoa, rinse it under cold water. Bring the water or vegetable broth to a boil in a saucepan. Reduce the heat to low, cover, and simmer for 15-20 minutes, or until

the quinoa is cooked and the liquid has been absorbed. Remove from the heat and set aside to cool.

3. Combine the chilled quinoa, diced cucumber, diced red bell pepper, finely sliced red onion, chopped parsley, and chopped mint leaves in a large mixing dish.

4. Whisk together the lemon juice, extra-virgin olive oil, salt, and pepper in a small bowl. Toss the quinoa salad with the dressing until completely combined. If necessary, adjust the seasoning. Set aside the salad.

5. Season both sides of the salmon fillets with salt and pepper. Place them, skin side down, on a hot grill. Grill the salmon for about 4-5 minutes per side, or until it's cooked through and flakes easily with a fork.

6. Remove the salmon from the grill and set it aside for a few minutes to rest.

7. Grilled salmon should be served atop a bed of quinoa salad. If preferred, garnish with more fresh herbs.

Baked Chicken Breast with Steamed Vegetables

Ingredients:

- 4 boneless, skinless chicken breasts
- 2 tablespoons olive oil
- 1 teaspoon garlic powder
- 1 teaspoon paprika
- 1/2 teaspoon salt
- 1/2 teaspoon black pepper
- 1 cup broccoli florets
- 1 cup cauliflower florets
- 1 cup carrot sticks
- 1 cup green beans, trimmed
- 2 tablespoons butter
- Salt and pepper to taste

Instructions:

1. Preheat the oven to 400 degrees Fahrenheit (200 degrees Celsius).
2. In a baking dish, sprinkle the chicken breasts with olive oil. Season with garlic powder, paprika, salt, and black pepper on both sides. Rub the ingredients into the chicken breasts with your hands.
3. Bake the chicken breasts for 20-25 minutes, or until they reach an internal temperature of 165°F (74°C) in a preheated oven. The cooking time will

depend on the thickness of the chicken breasts.

4. Prepare the steamed vegetables while the chicken is baking. Bring a big pot of water to a boil over high heat. Place a steamer basket or colander on top of the pot, but not in contact with the water.

5. Fill the steamer basket halfway with broccoli, cauliflower, carrots, and green beans. Cover with a lid and steam the vegetables for 5-7 minutes, or until soft but still crisp. Don't overcook them.

6. Remove the steamed veggies from the heat and place them in a serving bowl. Season with salt and pepper to taste after adding the butter. Gently toss until the butter melts and the vegetables are covered.

7. Remove the chicken breasts from the oven and set them aside for a few minutes to rest. This will aid in the retention of their fluids.

8. Thinly slice the baked chicken breasts diagonally.

9. Serve the cooked vegetables with the cut chicken breasts. If desired, garnish with fresh herbs such as parsley or basil.

Vegetable Stir-Fry with Tofu

Ingredients:

- 14 ounces (400g) firm tofu, drained and cubed
- 2 tablespoons soy sauce
- 1 tablespoon cornstarch
- 2 tablespoons vegetable oil
- 3 cloves garlic, minced
- 1 tablespoon ginger, grated
- 1 medium onion, sliced
- 2 medium carrots, julienned
- 1 bell pepper, thinly sliced
- 1 cup broccoli florets
- 1 cup snap peas, ends trimmed
- 1 cup mushrooms, sliced
- 2 tablespoons oyster sauce (optional for added flavor)
- 1 tablespoon sesame oil
- Salt and pepper to taste
- Cooked rice or noodles for serving

Instructions:

1. Combine the cubed tofu, soy sauce, and cornstarch in a mixing dish. Toss gently until the tofu is evenly coated. Allow to marinate for 10-15 minutes.
2. In a large skillet or wok, heat 1 tablespoon vegetable oil over medium-

high heat. Cook until the marinated tofu is golden brown and crispy on all sides. Set the tofu aside after removing it from the skillet.

3. Add the remaining tablespoon of vegetable oil to the same skillet. Sauté the minced garlic and grated ginger for about 1 minute, or until fragrant.
4. To the skillet, add the sliced onion, julienned carrots, bell pepper, broccoli florets, snap peas, and mushrooms. Stir-fry the vegetables for 5-7 minutes, or until crisp-tender.
5. Toss the tofu back into the skillet with the vegetables. If using, add the oyster sauce and sesame oil. Stir-fry for another 2-3 minutes, or until everything is fully mixed and thoroughly cooked.
6. Season to taste with salt and pepper. If desired, adjust the seasoning or add extra soy sauce.
7. Serve the tofu-vegetable stir-fry over cooked rice or noodles.

Turkey Meatballs with Zucchini Noodles

Ingredients:

- 1 pound ground turkey
- 1/2 cup breadcrumbs
- 1/4 cup grated Parmesan cheese
- 1/4 cup chopped fresh parsley
- 1/4 cup finely chopped onion
- 2 cloves garlic, minced
- 1 teaspoon dried oregano
- 1 teaspoon dried basil
- 1/2 teaspoon salt
- 1/4 teaspoon black pepper
- 2 large eggs
- 2 tablespoons olive oil
- 4-5 medium zucchini, spiralized into noodles
- 2 cups marinara sauce
- Fresh basil leaves, for garnish (optional)

Instructions:

1. Combine the ground turkey, breadcrumbs, Parmesan cheese, parsley, onion, garlic, oregano, basil, salt, black pepper, and eggs in a large mixing bowl. Mix until all of the ingredients are uniformly distributed.

2. Make small meatballs out of the turkey mixture, about 1 inch in diameter. You should obtain between 20 and 25 meatballs.

3. In a large skillet over medium heat, heat the olive oil. Cook the meatballs in the skillet for 8-10 minutes, rotating periodically, until browned and cooked through. Set the meatballs aside after removing them from the skillet.

4. In the same skillet, sauté the spiralized zucchini noodles for 2-3 minutes, or until they are slightly softened but still crunchy. Make sure not to overcook them or they will get mushy.

5. Stir the marinara sauce into the skillet with the zucchini noodles to mix. Return the cooked meatballs to the skillet and combine gently with the sauce and noodles. Allow everything to simmer for 2-3 minutes, or until the meatballs are well heated.

6. Serve the turkey meatballs and zucchini noodles on individual dishes. If desired, garnish with fresh basil leaves.

7. Enjoy the hot turkey meatballs with zucchini noodles!

Lentil Curry with Brown Rice

Ingredients:

- 1 cup brown lentils
- 1 cup brown rice
- 1 onion, finely chopped
- 2 garlic cloves, minced
- 1 tablespoon ginger, grated
- 1 tablespoon curry powder
- 1 teaspoon ground cumin
- 1 teaspoon ground coriander
- 1/2 teaspoon turmeric powder
- 1/2 teaspoon red chili powder (adjust to taste)
- 1 can (14 ounces) diced tomatoes
- 1 can (14 ounces) coconut milk
- 1 cup vegetable broth
- 2 tablespoons oil (such as olive or coconut oil)
- Salt to taste
- Fresh cilantro, chopped (for garnish)
- Lemon wedges (for serving)

Instructions:

1. Separately, rinse the lentils and brown rice in cold water. Place them aside.
2. In a big pot or Dutch oven, heat the oil over medium heat. Cook until the onions

have turned transparent, about 5 minutes. Stir every now and again.

3. To the pot, add the minced garlic and grated ginger. Cook for another minute, or until aromatic.

4. To the pot, add the curry powder, ground cumin, ground coriander, turmeric powder, and red chili powder. Stir in the spices to coat the onions, garlic, and ginger. To toast the spices, cook for about 1 minute.

5. To the pot, add the diced tomatoes (together with their liquids). Allow it to simmer for 2-3 minutes, stirring occasionally.

6. Pour in the rinsed lentils, coconut milk, and vegetable broth. Bring the mixture to a boil, stirring constantly.

7. Reduce the heat to low, cover, and leave to cook for 30-40 minutes, or until the lentils and rice are soft. To avoid sticking, stir occasionally.

8. Cook the brown rice according to package directions while the curry simmers. When it's done, fluff it with a fork.

9. When the lentils and rice are done, season the curry with salt to taste.

10. Serve the lentil curry with brown rice. Garnish with fresh cilantro and lemon juice if desired.

Grilled Shrimp Skewers with Roasted Sweet Potatoes

Ingredients:

- 1 pound of large shrimp, peeled and deveined
- 2 tablespoons of olive oil
- 2 cloves of garlic, minced
- 1 teaspoon of paprika
- 1 teaspoon of dried oregano
- 1/2 teaspoon of cayenne pepper (optional, for heat)
- Salt and pepper to taste
- 2 large sweet potatoes, peeled and cut into 1-inch cubes
- 2 tablespoons of melted butter
- Fresh parsley, chopped (for garnish)
- Wooden skewers, soaked in water for 30 minutes

Instructions:

1. Preheat the grill to medium-high.
2. Combine the olive oil, minced garlic, paprika, dried oregano, cayenne pepper (if using), salt, and pepper in a mixing bowl. Combine thoroughly.

3. Toss the shrimp in the basin with the marinade to coat evenly. Allow the shrimp to marinade for 15 minutes.
4. Preheat your oven to 400°F (200°C) in the meantime.
5. Toss the sweet potato cubes with the melted butter, salt, and pepper in a separate bowl.
6. On a baking sheet, arrange the sweet potato cubes in a single layer. Roast for 25-30 minutes, or until tender and slightly caramelized, in a preheated oven.
7. Thread the marinated shrimp onto the wooden skewers while the sweet potatoes cook.
8. Cook the shrimp skewers for about 2-3 minutes per side on a hot grill, or until the shrimp are pink and opaque.
9. Remove the shrimp from the grill and set them aside for a minute to rest.
10. Grilled shrimp skewers should be served atop roasted sweet potatoes. Garnish with parsley, if desired.

Quinoa Stuffed Bell Peppers

Ingredients:

- 4 bell peppers (any color)
- 1 cup quinoa, rinsed
- 2 cups vegetable broth

- 1 tablespoon olive oil
- 1 onion, diced
- 2 cloves garlic, minced
- 1 zucchini, diced
- 1 carrot, grated
- 1 cup canned black beans, drained and rinsed
- 1 cup corn kernels (fresh or frozen)
- 1 teaspoon ground cumin
- 1 teaspoon paprika
- 1/2 teaspoon chili powder
- Salt and pepper to taste
- 1/2 cup shredded cheddar cheese (optional)
- Fresh cilantro or parsley for garnish

Instructions:

1. Preheat the oven to 375 degrees Fahrenheit (190 degrees Celsius). Prepare a baking dish large enough to hold the bell peppers erect.
2. Remove the bell pepper tops and remove the seeds and membranes. Trim the bottoms slightly if necessary to help them stand upright in the baking dish. Place aside.
3. Bring the vegetable broth to a boil in a medium saucepan. Reduce the heat to low, cover, and cook for about 15

minutes, or until the quinoa is cooked and the liquid has been absorbed. Remove from the heat and let aside for 5 minutes, covered. Set aside after fluffing with a fork.

4. Warm the olive oil in a large skillet over medium heat. Sauté the diced onion and minced garlic for 3-4 minutes, or until the onion becomes transparent.
5. To the skillet, add the diced zucchini and shredded carrot. Cook for 5 minutes more, stirring periodically, until the vegetables are soft.
6. Add the cooked quinoa, black beans, corn kernels, cumin, paprika, chili powder, salt, and pepper to taste. Cook for another 2-3 minutes to enable the flavors to combine.
7. Pack the quinoa and veggie mixture tightly into the prepared bell peppers. Sprinkle some cheese on top of each stuffed pepper if using.
8. Place the stuffed bell peppers in the baking dish upright. You can use any leftover quinoa mixture to wrap around the peppers in the meal.
9. Bake for 25-30 minutes, or until the bell peppers are cooked, covered with foil.
10. Remove the foil and bake for 5 minutes further, or until the cheese (if used) is melted and slightly browned.

11. Remove the stuffed bell peppers from the oven and set aside for a few minutes to cool. Garnish with fresh cilantro or parsley if desired.

Baked Cod with Roasted Vegetables

Ingredients:

- 4 cod fillets
- 1 pound baby potatoes, halved
- 2 cups cherry tomatoes
- 1 red bell pepper, sliced
- 1 zucchini, sliced
- 1 red onion, cut into wedges
- 4 cloves of garlic, minced
- 2 tablespoons olive oil
- 1 teaspoon dried thyme
- 1 teaspoon dried rosemary
- Salt and pepper, to taste
- Fresh parsley, chopped (for garnish)

Instructions:

1. Preheat the oven to 400 degrees Fahrenheit (200 degrees Celsius).
2. Combine the split baby potatoes, cherry tomatoes, red bell pepper slices, zucchini slices, red onion wedges, minced garlic, olive oil, dried thyme, dried rosemary,

salt, and pepper in a large mixing dish. Toss all of the ingredients together until the veggies are fully coated with the oil and seasonings.

3. On a large baking sheet, equally distribute the seasoned vegetables. Cook for 20-25 minutes, or until the vegetables are soft and gently browned, on a baking sheet in a preheated oven. To ensure consistent roasting, stir the vegetables once or twice during the cooking process.

4. Prepare the fish fillets while the vegetables roast. Season the fillets on both sides with salt and pepper.

5. Remove the baking sheet from the oven after the vegetables have roasted for around 20 minutes. Make room for the cod fillets by pushing the roasted vegetables to one side of the baking pan.

6. Place the seasoned fish fillets on top of the roasted veggies on a baking sheet. Return the baking sheet to the oven for 10-12 minutes longer, or until the fish is cooked through and flakes readily with a fork.

7. Remove the fish and vegetables from the oven when they are done. Garnish with parsley, if desired.

8. Enjoy the delicious Baked Cod with Roasted Vegetables!

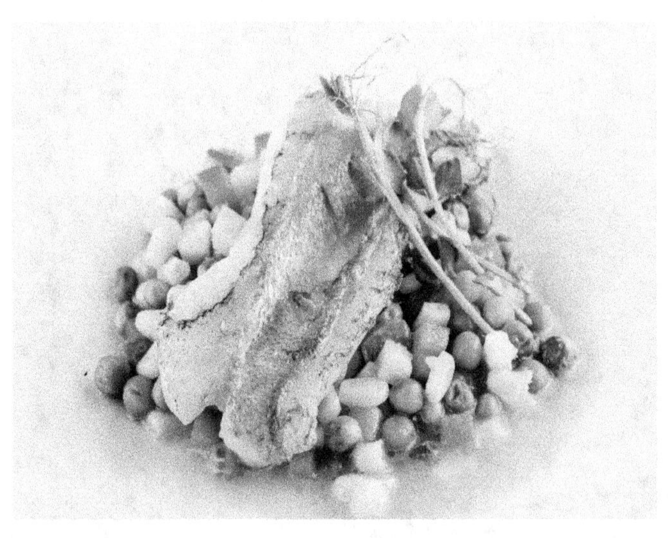

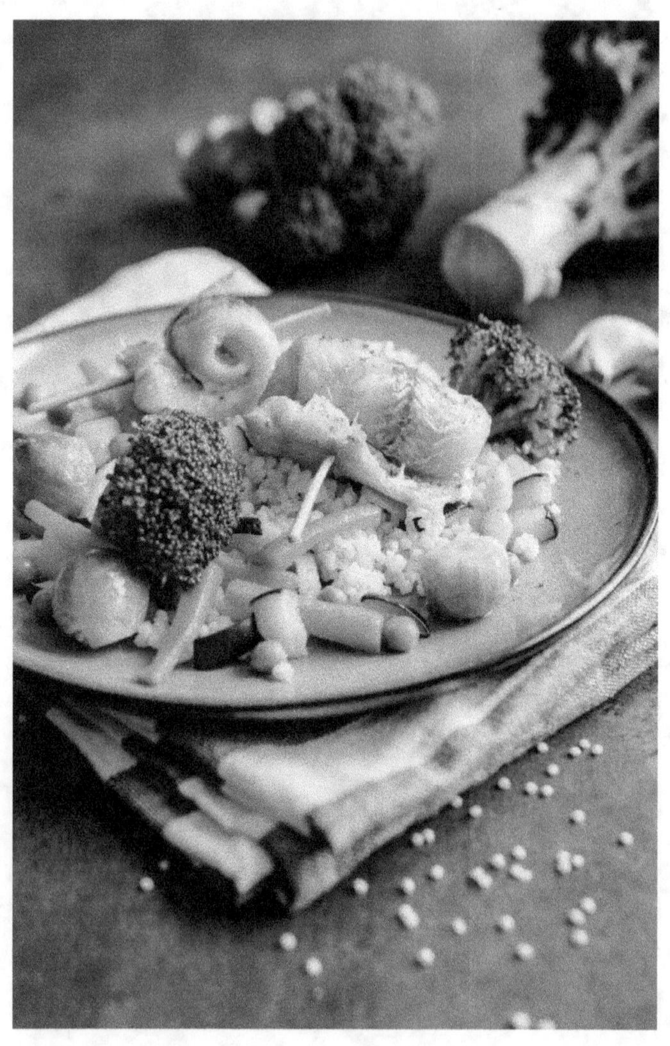

CHAPTER 4: APPETIZER AND SNACKS RECIPES

Veggie sticks with hummus dip

Ingredients:

For Veggie Sticks:

- Carrots
- Cucumbers
- Bell peppers (red, yellow, and/or green)
- Celery
- Cherry tomatoes
- For Hummus Dip:
-
- 1 can (15 ounces) chickpeas, drained and rinsed
- 2 cloves garlic, minced
- 3 tablespoons tahini
- 3 tablespoons freshly squeezed lemon juice
- 2 tablespoons olive oil
- 1/2 teaspoon ground cumin
- Salt and pepper to taste
- Water (as needed for consistency)
- Optional toppings: paprika, chopped parsley, drizzle of olive oil

Quinoa salad bites

Ingredients:
- For Veggie Sticks:
-
- Carrots
- Cucumbers
- Bell peppers (red, yellow, and/or green)
- Celery
- Cherry tomatoes
- For Hummus Dip:
-
- 1 can (15 ounces) chickpeas, drained and rinsed
- 2 cloves garlic, minced
- 3 tablespoons tahini
- 3 tablespoons freshly squeezed lemon juice
- 2 tablespoons olive oil
- 1/2 teaspoon ground cumin
- Salt and pepper to taste
- Water (as needed for consistency)
- Optional toppings: paprika, chopped parsley, drizzle of olive oil

Instructions:

1. Make the vegetable sticks:
2. Peel and wash the carrots. Cut them into finger-length sticks that are thin.
3. Cucumbers should be washed before being cut into long, thin strips.
4. Bell peppers should have their seeds and stem removed before being chopped into small strips.
5. After cleaning, slice celery into sticks.
6. Wash cherry tomatoes.
7. How to make hummus dip:
8. The chickpeas, minced garlic, tahini, lemon juice, olive oil, cumin, salt, and pepper should all be combined in a food processor or blender.
9. Blend the ingredients thoroughly. If it's too thick, add water a tablespoon at a time until the appropriate consistency is achieved.
10. When necessary, taste and adjust the seasonings.
11. Build and Serve:
12. Place the veggie sticks on individual plates or a serving dish.
13. Put a dish of the hummus dip in the middle or on one of the platter's sides.
14. You may also drizzle some olive oil over the hummus and top it with some paprika and chopped parsley.
15. Enjoy the Veggie Sticks and Hummus Dip together!

Greek yogurt with berries

Ingredients:

- 1 cup Greek yogurt
- 1 cup mixed berries (such as strawberries, blueberries, raspberries)
- 1 tablespoon honey (optional)
- 2 tablespoons granola (optional)

Instructions:

1. Wash and wipe dry the berries completely. Remove the stems from the strawberries and cut them into bite-sized pieces.
2. Combine the Greek yogurt and honey (if using) in a mixing dish. Mix until the honey is equally distributed throughout the yogurt.
3. Fold the mixed berries into the yogurt carefully to ensure they are well distributed.
4. Sprinkle granola on top of the yogurt and berries if preferred for crunch and texture.
5. Enjoy the Greek yogurt with berries right away!

Cucumber and cream cheese roll-ups

Ingredients:

- 4 large cucumbers
- 8 ounces (225 grams) cream cheese, softened
- 1 tablespoon fresh dill, finely chopped
- 1 tablespoon fresh chives, finely chopped
- Salt and pepper to taste

Instructions:

1. Wash the cucumbers thoroughly and cut the ends off. Peel long, thin strips from each cucumber using a vegetable peeler, discarding the first strip (which will primarily be the peel). Continue peeling until each cucumber has a strip.
2. Combine the softened cream cheese, fresh dill, and fresh chives in a mixing dish. Season to taste with salt and pepper. Mix until all of the ingredients are uniformly distributed.
3. Place the cucumber slices on a clean surface. Cover each strip completely with a thin layer of the cream cheese mixture.
4. Begin rolling up each cucumber strip from one end, making sure the cream cheese is securely wrapped within.

Recycle the cucumber strips and cream cheese mixture as needed.

5. Place the cucumber roll-ups on a serving dish or plate once they are finished. If required, fasten them with toothpicks.

6. Refrigerate the roll-ups for about 30 minutes before serving for the best results. This allows them to firm up and the flavors to blend.

7. As an appetizer or snack, serve chilled. Enjoy the cool crunch of cucumber with the creamy, herb-infused cream cheese filling

Roasted chickpeas

Ingredients:

- 2 cans (15 ounces each) of chickpeas (garbanzo beans)
- 2 tablespoons olive oil
- 1 teaspoon ground cumin
- 1 teaspoon paprika
- 1/2 teaspoon garlic powder
- 1/2 teaspoon onion powder
- 1/2 teaspoon salt (adjust to taste)
- 1/4 teaspoon black pepper
- Optional: pinch of cayenne pepper for some heat
- Fresh parsley or cilantro (for garnish)

Instructions:

1. Preheat the oven to 400 degrees Fahrenheit (200 degrees Celsius). To make cleanup easier, line a baking pan with parchment paper or aluminum foil.
2. In a colander, drain and rinse the chickpeas. Using a clean kitchen towel or paper towels, pat them dry. Remove any loose skins that may have fallen off during the rinsing process.
3. Combine the chickpeas, olive oil, cumin, paprika, garlic powder, onion powder, salt, black pepper, and cayenne pepper (if using) in a mixing bowl. Toss well to coat all of the chickpeas with the spice mixture.
4. On the prepared baking sheet, spread the seasoned chickpeas in a single layer. To ensure consistent roasting, make sure they are properly spaced.
5. Roast the chickpeas on a baking sheet in a preheated oven for 25-30 minutes, or until golden brown and crispy. To ensure even browning, gently shake the baking sheet or stir the chickpeas halfway during the cooking time.
6. Remove the chickpeas from the oven and set them aside to cool for a few minutes

on the baking sheet. As they cool, they will continue to crisp up.

7. Put the roasted chickpeas in a serving basin. If preferred, garnish with fresh parsley or cilantro.

8. Serve the roasted chickpeas alone as a snack or as a crispy topping for salads, soups, or roasted vegetable bowls. Enjoy!

Avocado and tomato bruschetta

Ingredients:

- 1 large ripe avocado
- 2 medium tomatoes
- 1 small red onion
- 2 cloves of garlic
- 1 tablespoon fresh lemon juice
- 2 tablespoons fresh basil leaves, chopped
- Salt and black pepper to taste
- 1 baguette or Italian bread loaf
- Olive oil for drizzling

Instructions:

1. Preheat the oven to 375 degrees Fahrenheit (190 degrees Celsius). Place the baguette on a baking sheet and slice it into 1/2-inch thick slices. Drizzle the bread pieces with olive oil.

2. Bake the bread pieces in a preheated oven for 8-10 minutes, or until toasted and golden brown. Set aside to cool after removing from the oven.
3. Prepare the avocado and tomato mixture while the bread is browning. Remove the pit from the avocado and scoop out the flesh into a medium-sized bowl. With a fork, mash the avocado until it reaches the required consistency.
4. Chop the red onion and garlic cloves coarsely and dice the tomatoes. Combine them with the mashed avocado in a mixing dish.
5. To the bowl, add the fresh lemon juice, basil leaves, salt, and black pepper. Mix all of the ingredients until completely blended.
6. Adjust the seasoning to taste with the avocado and tomato mixture.
7. Once the toasted bread pieces have cooled slightly, dollop the avocado and tomato mixture evenly onto each slice.
8. Enjoy the avocado and tomato bruschetta right away!

Spinach and feta stuffed mushrooms

Ingredients:

- 12 large mushrooms (cremini or button mushrooms work well)
- 1 tablespoon olive oil
- 1 small onion, finely chopped
- 2 cloves garlic, minced
- 2 cups fresh spinach, chopped
- 1/2 cup crumbled feta cheese
- 1/4 cup grated Parmesan cheese
- 1/4 cup breadcrumbs
- 1/4 teaspoon dried oregano
- Salt and pepper to taste
- Fresh parsley, chopped (for garnish)

Instructions:

1. Preheat the oven to 375 degrees Fahrenheit (190 degrees Celsius). Set aside a baking dish that has been lightly greased.
2. Remove the mushroom stems and coarsely slice them. Set aside the mushroom caps.
3. In a large skillet over medium heat, heat the olive oil. Sauté the chopped onion and minced garlic until they are tender and transparent.
4. Cook for an additional 3-4 minutes, or until the mushroom stems shed their moisture, in the skillet.

5. Cook, stirring constantly, until the spinach wilts and any extra moisture evaporates. Take the pan off the heat.
6. Combine the cooked spinach mixture, crumbled feta cheese, grated Parmesan cheese, breadcrumbs, dried oregano, salt, and pepper in a mixing bowl. Mix everything together until everything is uniformly   distrib

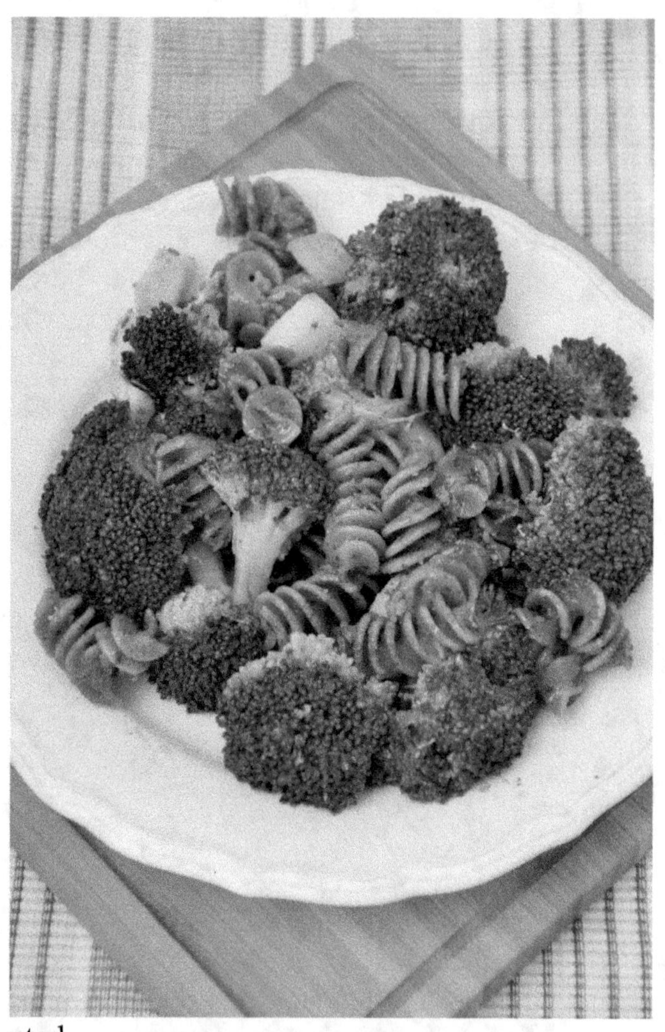

uted.

7. Fill the mushroom caps with the filling, gently pressing it down. Place the stuffed mushrooms in the baking dish that has been prepared.

8. Bake the stuffed mushrooms for 20-25 minutes, or until the mushrooms are soft and the filling is brown and bubbling in a preheated oven.
9. Remove from the oven and set aside to cool. Before serving, garnish with freshly cut parsley.

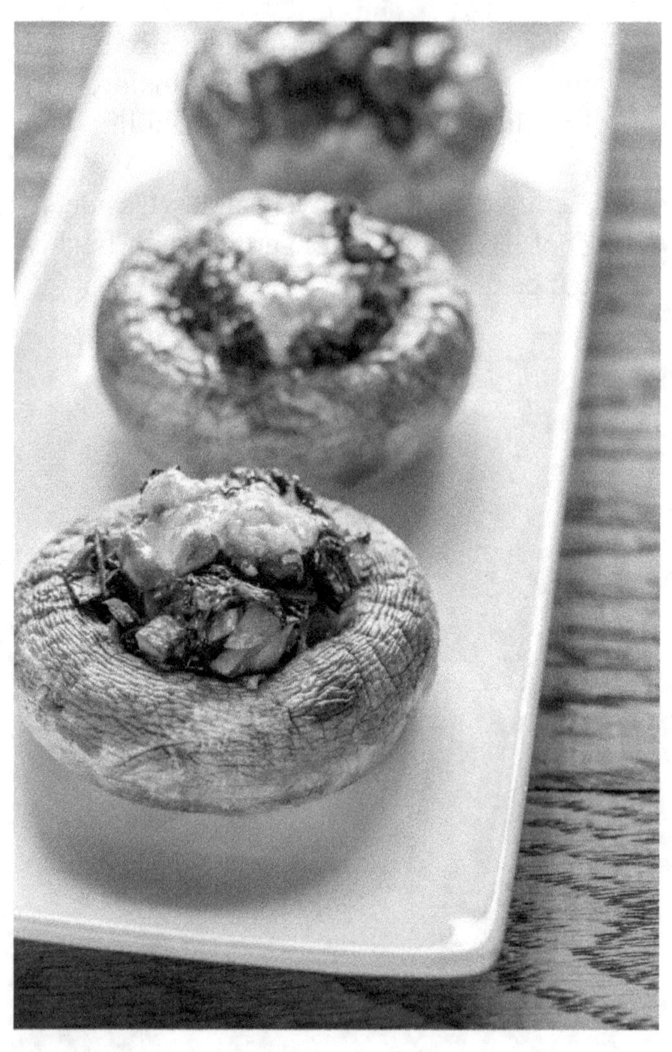

CHAPTER 5: SOUPS AND SALADS

Ingredients:

- 2 pounds of ripe tomatoes
- 1 large onion, chopped
- 4 cloves of garlic, minced
- 1 tablespoon of olive oil
- 4 cups of vegetable or chicken broth
- 1 cup of fresh basil leaves, chopped
- 1 teaspoon of sugar
- Salt and pepper to taste
- Optional: 1/2 cup of heavy cream or coconut milk for added creaminess

Instructions:

1. Begin by chopping the tomatoes. Bring a kettle of water to a boil and cut a little "X" in the bottom of each tomato. Place the tomatoes in a bowl of ice water after about 30 seconds in the boiling water. This procedure will aid in the removal of the skin. Peel and roughly slice the tomatoes.

2. Warm the olive oil in a large soup pot over medium heat. Sauté the chopped onion and minced garlic for 5 minutes, or until tender and transparent.
3. Cook for another 5 minutes, stirring regularly, with the chopped tomatoes and any fluids that have gathered in the saucepan.
4. Bring the mixture to a boil with the vegetable or chicken broth. Reduce the heat to low, cover the pot, and allow it to simmer for about 20 minutes to enable the flavors to blend.
5. Remove the saucepan from the heat and set aside for a few minutes to allow the soup to cool. Puree the soup with an immersion blender or a tabletop blender until smooth. To avoid overfilling a countertop blender, proceed in batches.
6. Return the soup to the pot and cook it on low. Add the basil leaves, sugar, salt, and pepper to taste. For extra richness, add the optional heavy cream or coconut milk. Continue to heat the soup for 5 minutes, stirring regularly.
7. Adjust the seasonings to your liking after tasting the soup.
8. When the soup has been thoroughly heated and seasoned to your desire, it is ready to serve. Pour the tomato and basil soup into dishes and top with fresh basil

leaves. To add more taste, pour some olive oil on top.

Lentil soup

Ingredients:

- 1 cup dried lentils
- 1 onion, diced
- 2 carrots, diced
- 2 celery stalks, diced
- 3 cloves of garlic, minced
- 1 can diced tomatoes
- 4 cups vegetable broth
- 1 teaspoon ground cumin
- 1 teaspoon ground coriander
- 1/2 teaspoon smoked paprika
- Salt and pepper to taste
- 2 tablespoons olive oil
- Fresh cilantro or parsley, chopped (for garnish)

Instructions:

1. Remove any debris or stones by rinsing the lentils under cold water. Place aside.
2. In a large pot or Dutch oven, heat the olive oil over medium heat. Combine the onion, carrots, and celery in a mixing

bowl. Cook for 5 minutes, or until the vegetables soften.

3. To the pot, add the minced garlic, cumin, coriander, smoked paprika, salt, and pepper. Cook for an additional minute after thoroughly coating the vegetables with the seasonings.

4. To the pot, add the lentils, diced tomatoes (with juice), and vegetable broth. Bring the water to a boil.

5. Reduce the heat to low and cover the pot after it begins to boil. Cook for 30-40 minutes, or until the lentils are cooked.

6. If desired, mix a portion of the soup with an immersion blender to achieve a thicker consistency. Alternatively, puree a cup or two of the soup in a blender before returning it to the saucepan.

7. Adjust the seasonings as needed after tasting the soup.

8. Serve the lentil soup hot with fresh cilantro or parsley on top. If desired, pour some lemon juice over the soup for an added acidic flavor.

Butternut squash soup

Ingredients:

- 1 large butternut squash

- 1 tablespoon olive oil
- 1 medium onion, chopped
- 2 cloves garlic, minced
- 4 cups vegetable broth
- 1 teaspoon ground cumin
- 1/2 teaspoon ground cinnamon
- 1/4 teaspoon ground nutmeg
- Salt and pepper to taste
- 1/2 cup heavy cream (optional, for added creaminess)
- Fresh parsley or chives for garnish

Instructions:

1. Preheat the oven to 400 degrees Fahrenheit (200 degrees Celsius). Scoop out the seeds after cutting the butternut squash in half lengthwise. Place the squash halves, cut side up, on a baking sheet. Drizzle with olive oil and season with salt and pepper to taste. Cook for about 45 minutes, or until the flesh is fork-tender.
2. Remove the squash from the oven and set aside to cool slightly. Scoop out the flesh with a spoon and set it aside.
3. Warm the olive oil in a big pot over medium heat. Sauté the chopped onion and garlic for 5 minutes, or until transparent and aromatic.

4. Add the roasted butternut squash flesh, vegetable broth, ground cumin, ground cinnamon, and ground nutmeg to the pot. To blend, stir everything together thoroughly. Bring the mixture to a boil, then reduce to a low heat, cover, and leave to simmer for about 15 minutes to enable the flavors to blend.

5. After simmering, mix the soup with an immersion blender or in stages in a countertop blender until smooth and creamy. When blending hot liquids with a countertop blender, use caution. Keep a vent open to allow steam to escape.

6. Return the pureed soup to the pot and cook on low. If using, stir in the heavy cream and season with salt and pepper to taste. Allow the soup to heat thoroughly without boiling it.

7. Remove the soup from the heat once it has heated through. Pour into serving bowls and top with fresh parsley or chives.

Minestrone soup

Ingredients:

- 2 tablespoons olive oil
- 1 medium onion, diced

- 2 cloves garlic, minced
- 2 carrots, diced
- 2 celery stalks, diced
- 1 zucchini, diced
- 1 cup green beans, cut into 1-inch pieces
- 1 can (14 ounces) diced tomatoes
- 4 cups vegetable broth
- 2 cups water
- 1 teaspoon dried basil
- 1 teaspoon dried oregano
- 1/2 teaspoon dried thyme
- 1/2 teaspoon salt (adjust to taste)
- 1/4 teaspoon black pepper
- 1 can (15 ounces) cannellini beans, drained and rinsed
- 1 cup small pasta (such as macaroni or shells)
- 2 cups fresh spinach, chopped
- Grated Parmesan cheese, for serving

Instructions:

1. In a large pot over medium heat, heat the olive oil. Sauté the onion and garlic until they are aromatic and transparent.
2. Toss in the carrots, celery, zucchini, and green beans. Cook, stirring occasionally, for about 5 minutes, or until the vegetables begin to soften.
3. Combine the diced tomatoes, vegetable broth, and water in a mixing bowl. Add

the dried basil, oregano, thyme, salt, and black pepper to taste. Bring the ingredients to a boil.

4. Reduce the heat to low and continue to cook the soup for 20 minutes, or until the veggies are soft.
5. Pour in the cannellini beans and pasta. Cook for 10 minutes more, or until the pasta is al dente.
6. Cook for an additional 2 minutes, or until the spinach wilts, after adding the chopped spinach.
7. If necessary, taste the soup and adjust the seasoning.
8. Turn off the heat in the pot. Garnish the Minestrone soup with grated Parmesan cheese and serve immediately.

Chicken and vegetable soup

Ingredients:

- 1 tablespoon olive oil
- 1 onion, diced
- 2 cloves garlic, minced
- 2 carrots, peeled and sliced
- 2 celery stalks, sliced
- 1 red bell pepper, diced
- 4 cups chicken broth
- 2 cups cooked chicken, shredded or diced

- 1 cup frozen corn kernels
- 1 cup frozen peas
- 1 teaspoon dried thyme
- 1 bay leaf
- Salt and pepper to taste
- Fresh parsley, chopped (for garnish)

Instructions:

1. In a large pot over medium heat, heat the olive oil. Sauté the diced onion and minced garlic until the onion is transparent and aromatic.
2. To the pot, add the sliced carrots, celery, and diced red bell pepper. Cook, stirring occasionally, for about 5 minutes, or until the vegetables begin to soften.
3. Bring the mixture to a boil by adding the chicken broth. Reduce the heat to low and allow the flavors to combine for 10 minutes.
4. To the pot, add the cooked chicken, frozen corn kernels, frozen peas, dried thyme, and bay leaf. To blend, stir everything together thoroughly.
5. Cook for another 10-15 minutes, or until the veggies are soft and the flavors have formed. Season to taste with salt and pepper.

6. Remove the bay leaf from the saucepan and set it aside.
7. Serve the chicken and vegetable soup hot with fresh chopped parsley on top.

Broccoli and cheddar soup

Ingredients:

- 2 tablespoons butter
- 1 medium onion, chopped
- 2 cloves garlic, minced
- 4 cups broccoli florets
- 3 cups chicken or vegetable broth
- 1 cup milk
- 1 cup shredded cheddar cheese
- Salt and pepper to taste

Instructions:

1. Melt the butter in a big pot over medium heat. Cook, stirring frequently, until the onion and garlic are tender and transparent, about 5 minutes.
2. Stir in the broccoli florets along with the onions and garlic. Cook for another 2-3 minutes to soften the broccoli slightly.
3. Bring the mixture to a boil with the chicken or veggie broth. Reduce the heat

to low, cover the saucepan, and cook for 15-20 minutes, or until the broccoli is cooked.

4. Puree the soup with an immersion blender or a conventional blender until smooth. When mixing hot liquids, use caution and work in batches if using a normal blender.

5. Stir in the milk and return the soup to the pot. Warm the soup gently over low heat, but do not allow it to boil.

6. Add the shredded cheddar cheese to the soup gradually, swirling frequently, until it melts and blends in. This will result in a creamy, cheesy feel.

7. Season the soup to taste with salt and pepper. Seasoning can be adjusted to your liking.

8. Remove the soup from the heat once the cheese has completely melted and it is well cooked.

9. Serve the broccoli and cheddar soup in bowls, heated. If desired, top with more shredded cheese or chopped fresh herbs.

Spinach and white bean soup

Ingredients:

- 1 tablespoon olive oil
- 1 medium onion, diced

- 3 cloves garlic, minced
- 2 carrots, diced
- 2 celery stalks, diced
- 4 cups vegetable broth
- 2 cans (15 ounces each) white beans, drained and rinsed
- 1 can (14 ounces) diced tomatoes
- 1 teaspoon dried thyme
- 1 bay leaf
- 4 cups fresh spinach leaves
- Salt and pepper to taste
- Grated Parmesan cheese for garnish (optional)

Instructions:

1. In a large pot over medium heat, heat the olive oil. Sauté the diced onion and minced garlic for 5 minutes, or until the onion becomes translucent and fragrant.
2. Cook for another 5 minutes, or until the carrots and celery start to soften, in the pot with the diced carrots and celery.
3. Pour in the vegetable broth, white beans, and tomato diced with juice. Combine the dried thyme and bay leaf in a mixing bowl. Bring the soup to a boil, then reduce to a low heat and allow it to simmer for about 20 minutes to enable the flavors to blend.

4. Remove the bay leaf from the saucepan and set it aside. Puree roughly half of the soup using an immersion blender or a standard blender to make a creamy base. Alternatively, for a chunkier texture, lightly mash part of the beans and vegetables using a potato masher.

5. Return the soup to a low heat and stir in the spinach leaves. Stir gently for 2-3 minutes, or until the spinach wilts and turns soft.

6. Season the soup to taste with salt and pepper. Keep in mind to taste and adjust the seasoning as needed.

7. Serve the spinach and white bean soup hot in bowls. Garnish each plate with grated Parmesan cheese, if preferred.

Carrot ginger soup

Ingredients:

- 1 tablespoon olive oil
- 1 medium onion, diced
- 3 cloves garlic, minced
- 1 tablespoon fresh ginger, grated
- 4 cups carrots, peeled and chopped
- 4 cups vegetable broth
- 1 cup coconut milk
- 1 teaspoon ground cumin

- 1/2 teaspoon ground coriander
- Salt and pepper to taste
- Fresh cilantro or parsley for garnish (optional)

Instructions:

1. In a large pot over medium heat, heat the olive oil. Combine the diced onion, minced garlic, and grated ginger in a mixing bowl. Cook for 5 minutes, or until the onion is transparent and the ginger is fragrant.
2. Stir in the chopped carrots to coat them in the onion-ginger mixture. Cook for another 5 minutes to soften the vegetables slightly.
3. Bring the mixture to a boil with the vegetable broth. Reduce to a low heat and cook for 15-20 minutes, or until the carrots are soft and easily penetrated with a fork.
4. Puree the soup with an immersion blender or a conventional blender until smooth and creamy. When mixing hot liquids, use caution and work in batches if using a normal blender.
5. Return the pureed soup to the pot and cook on low. Combine the coconut milk,

cumin, and coriander in a mixing bowl.
Allow the soup to simmer for 5 minutes
more to combine the flavors.

6. Season the soup to taste with salt and
   pepper. Seasoning can be adjusted to your
   liking.

7. Ladle the carrot ginger soup into dishes
   and, if preferred, garnish with fresh
   cilantro or parsley.

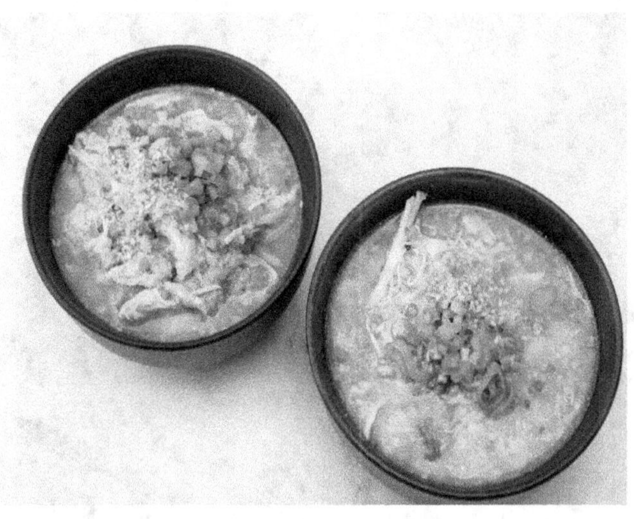

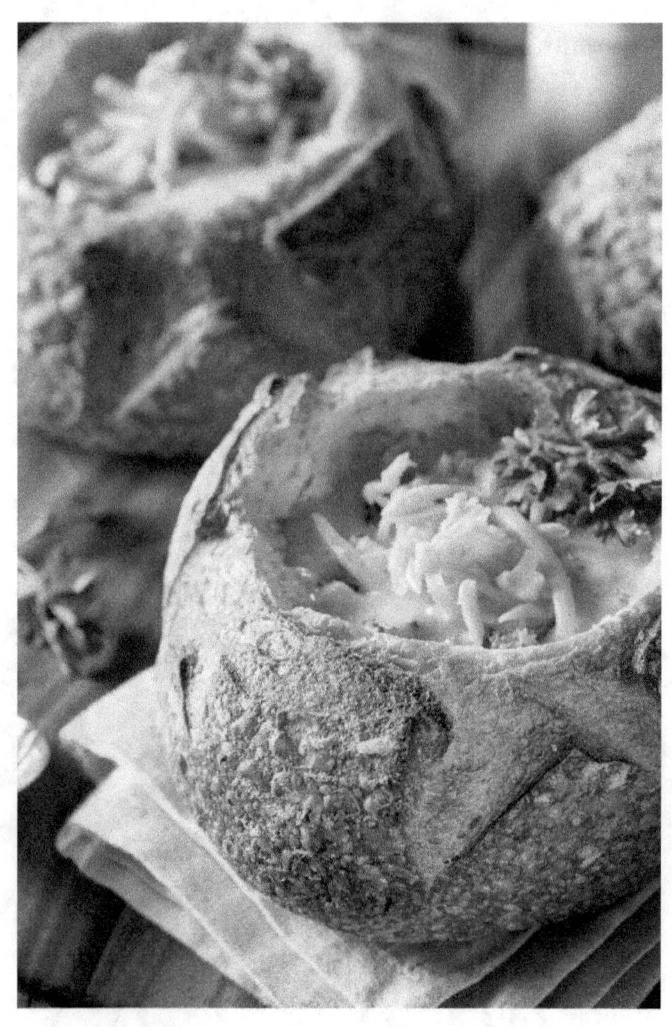

CHAPTER 6: MAIN DISHES

roasted salmon with turmeric

Ingredients:

- 4 salmon fillets
- 1 tablespoon turmeric powder
- 1 teaspoon paprika
- 1 teaspoon garlic powder
- 1 teaspoon salt
- 1/2 teaspoon black pepper
- 2 tablespoons olive oil
- Fresh lemon wedges, for serving
- Chopped fresh parsley, for garnish

Instructions:

1. Preheat the oven to 400°F (200°C) and line or lightly butter a baking sheet with parchment paper.
2. Combine the turmeric powder, paprika, garlic powder, salt, and black pepper in a small bowl. To make a spice rub, thoroughly combine all of the ingredients.
3. Place the salmon fillets on the baking sheet that has been prepared. Drizzle the

olive oil evenly over the fillets, then sprinkle with the spice rub, coating all sides.

4. Gently rub the spices into the salmon fillets to coat them evenly. Allow the salmon to marinade for about 15 minutes at room temperature, or up to 1 hour in the refrigerator for a stronger taste.

5. Place the baking sheet with the salmon in the preheated oven once it has been marinated. Cook for 12-15 minutes, or until the salmon is cooked through and easily flakes with a fork.

6. Remove the salmon from the oven and set aside for a few minutes to rest. The liquids will redistribute and the flavors will mix as a result of this.

7. Serve the turmeric-roasted salmon with fresh lemon wedges for squeezing over the top. To add freshness and color, garnish with chopped fresh parsley.

Grilled chicken breast with roasted vegetables

Ingredients:

- 2 boneless, skinless chicken breasts
- 2 tablespoons olive oil

- 2 cloves garlic, minced
- 1 teaspoon paprika
- 1 teaspoon dried oregano
- 1/2 teaspoon salt
- 1/4 teaspoon black pepper
- 1 large zucchini, sliced
- 1 red bell pepper, sliced
- 1 yellow bell pepper, sliced
- 1 red onion, sliced
- 1 tablespoon balsamic vinegar
- Fresh parsley, chopped (for garnish)

Instructions:

1. Preheat the grill to medium-high.
2. To make the marinade for the chicken, combine 1 tablespoon olive oil, minced garlic, paprika, dried oregano, salt, and black pepper in a small bowl.
3. Pour the marinade over the chicken breasts in a ziplock bag or shallow dish. Make sure the chicken is evenly coated with the marinade. Allow the chicken to marinade at room temperature for about 20 minutes.
4. Preheat the oven to 425°F (220°C) as the chicken marinates.
5. Combine the sliced zucchini, red and yellow bell peppers, and red onion in a large mixing basin. Drizzle with 1 tablespoon olive oil and 1 tablespoon

balsamic vinegar. Toss the vegetables in the dressing until evenly coated.

6. Arrange the vegetables on a baking sheet lined with parchment paper in a single layer. Roast the vegetables in a warm oven for 20-25 minutes, or until soft and slightly browned, tossing halfway through.

7. While the veggies roast, grill the chicken breasts for 6-8 minutes per side on a hot grill, or until the internal temperature reaches 165°F (74°C). The cooking time will vary according to the thickness of the chicken breasts.

8. Remove the chicken from the grill and let it rest for a few minutes before slicing it into strips.

9. Arrange the grilled chicken slices on a serving plate, followed by the roasted veggies. Garnish with fresh parsley if desired.

10. As a delicious and healthful main course, serve the grilled chicken breast with roasted veggies.

Ingredients:

1. 1 pound (450g) shrimp, peeled and deveined
2. 2 tablespoons vegetable oil, divided
3. 3 cloves garlic, minced
4. 1-inch piece of ginger, grated
5. 1 red bell pepper, sliced
6. 1 yellow bell pepper, sliced
7. 1 medium carrot, julienned
8. 1 cup broccoli florets
9. 1 cup snap peas, ends trimmed
10. 1 cup sliced mushrooms
11. 2 tablespoons soy sauce
12. 1 tablespoon oyster sauce
13. 1 tablespoon hoisin sauce
14. 1 teaspoon sesame oil
15. 1/4 teaspoon red pepper flakes (optional)
16. Salt and pepper, to taste
17. Fresh cilantro or green onions for garnish

Instructions:

1. Heat 1 tablespoon vegetable oil in a large skillet or wok over medium-high heat.
2. Stir-fry the shrimp in the skillet for 2-3 minutes, or until they turn pink and opaque. Take the shrimp out of the skillet and set aside.

3. Add the remaining tablespoon of vegetable oil to the same skillet. Stir in the minced garlic and grated ginger for about 1 minute, or until fragrant.
4. To the skillet, add the sliced bell peppers, julienned carrot, broccoli florets, snap peas, and sliced mushrooms. 3-4 minutes, or until the vegetables are crisp-tender.
5. Whisk together the soy sauce, oyster sauce, hoisin sauce, sesame oil, and red pepper flakes (if using) in a small bowl.
6. Return the cooked shrimp and vegetables to the skillet. Serve the shrimp and vegetables with the sauce mixture. Stir-fry for another 1-2 minutes to evenly coat everything. Season to taste with salt and pepper.
7. Turn off the heat in the skillet. Serve the shrimp stir-fry garnished with fresh cilantro or green onions.
8. Over steaming rice or noodles, serve the shrimp stir-fry with mixed vegetables.

Turkey meatballs with zucchini noodles

Ingredients:

- 1 pound ground turkey
- 1/2 cup breadcrumbs
- 1/4 cup grated Parmesan cheese

- 1/4 cup chopped fresh parsley
- 2 cloves garlic, minced
- 1 teaspoon dried oregano
- 1/2 teaspoon salt
- 1/4 teaspoon black pepper
- 2 large eggs
- 2 tablespoons olive oil
- 4 medium zucchini
- 2 cups marinara sauce
- Fresh basil leaves, for garnish (optional)

Instructions:

1. Combine ground turkey, breadcrumbs, Parmesan cheese, parsley, minced garlic, dried oregano, salt, black pepper, and eggs in a large mixing basin. Mix until all of the ingredients are uniformly distributed.
2. Form the turkey mixture into 1 to 1 1/2-inch-diameter meatballs. Place aside.
3. In a large skillet over medium heat, heat the olive oil. Cook until the meatballs are browned on all sides, about 8-10 minutes. Check that the meatballs are cooked through by cutting one open.
4. Prepare the zucchini noodles while the meatballs are cooking. Trim the ends of the zucchini and produce long, thin noodles with a spiralizer or julienne peeler. Alternatively, you can make

broader ribbon-like noodles with a vegetable peeler.

5. Remove the meatballs from the skillet and set aside after cooked. Sauté the zucchini noodles in the same skillet for 2-3 minutes, or until they are just soft.

6. Stir the marinara sauce into the zucchini noodles in the skillet to coat them evenly. Cook for another 2-3 minutes to allow the sauce to heat through.

7. Return the meatballs, zucchini noodles, and sauce to the skillet. Toss everything together gently until the meatballs and noodles are coated in sauce and heated completely.

8. In bowls or on plates, serve the turkey meatballs and zucchini noodles. If desired, garnish with fresh basil leaves.

Baked cod with cherry tomatoes and olives

Ingredients:

- 4 cod fillets
- 2 cups cherry tomatoes, halved
- 1 cup pitted black olives
- 4 cloves garlic, minced
- 2 tablespoons fresh basil, chopped

- 2 tablespoons fresh parsley, chopped
- 2 tablespoons olive oil
- 1 lemon, sliced
- Salt and pepper to taste

Instructions:

1. Preheat the oven to 400 degrees Fahrenheit (200 degrees Celsius).
2. Drizzle 1 tablespoon olive oil in a baking dish. Coat the bottom of the dish evenly with it.
3. In the baking dish, arrange the fish fillets. Season with salt and pepper to taste.
4. Combine the cherry tomatoes, black olives, minced garlic, chopped basil, and parsley in a mixing bowl. Gently toss them together.
5. Distribute the tomato and olive mixture equally over the fish fillets.
6. Drizzle the fish and veggies with the remaining tablespoon of olive oil.
7. Serve the cod fillets with lemon slices on top.
8. Cover the baking dish with foil and bake for 15-20 minutes, or until the fish is opaque and readily flaked with a fork.
9. Remove the foil and continue to broil for another 2-3 minutes to lightly brown the top.

10. Remove the baking dish from the oven with care. Serve the baked cod with cherry tomatoes and olives hot, topped if preferred with fresh basil or parsley.

Vegetable curry with brown rice

Ingredients:

- 1 cup brown rice
- 2 tablespoons vegetable oil
- 1 onion, diced
- 3 garlic cloves, minced
- 1-inch piece of ginger, grated
- 2 carrots, sliced
- 1 bell pepper, diced
- 1 small cauliflower, cut into florets
- 1 zucchini, sliced
- 1 cup green beans, trimmed and cut into bite-sized pieces
- 1 can (14 ounces) coconut milk
- 2 tablespoons curry powder
- 1 teaspoon turmeric powder
- 1 teaspoon cumin powder
- 1 teaspoon coriander powder
- Salt to taste
- Fresh cilantro leaves, for garnish

Instructions:

1. Brown rice should be cooked according to package directions. Place aside.
2. In a large pot or skillet, heat the vegetable oil over medium heat. Sauté the sliced onion until it gets transparent.
3. Cook for another minute, stirring regularly to prevent scorching, after adding the minced garlic and grated ginger to the pot.
4. To the pot, add the carrots, bell pepper, cauliflower, zucchini, and green beans. For a few minutes, stir-fry the vegetables until they begin to soften.
5. Combine the curry powder, turmeric powder, cumin powder, and coriander powder in a small bowl. Stir the spice mixture into the pot to coat the vegetables.
6. Pour in the coconut milk and mix well. Bring the mixture to a boil, then lower to a low heat. Allow the curry to simmer for 15-20 minutes, or until the vegetables are soft.
7. Season the curry with salt to taste.
8. Serve the vegetable curry with brown rice. Garnish with fresh cilantro leaves if desired.

Lean beef stir-fry with broccoli and ginger

Ingredients:

- 1 pound lean beef, sliced into thin strips
- 2 cups broccoli florets
- 1 tablespoon fresh ginger, minced
- 3 cloves garlic, minced
- 2 tablespoons low-sodium soy sauce
- 1 tablespoon oyster sauce
- 1 tablespoon cornstarch
- 2 tablespoons vegetable oil
- Salt and pepper to taste
- Cooked rice, for serving

Instructions:

1. Combine the soy sauce, oyster sauce, and cornstarch in a small bowl. Place aside.
2. In a large skillet or wok, heat 1 tablespoon vegetable oil over medium-high heat.
3. Stir-fry the sliced beef in the skillet for 3-4 minutes, or until browned and cooked through. Set the steak aside after removing it from the skillet.
4. Add the remaining tablespoon of vegetable oil to the same skillet.

5. Stir-fry the minced ginger and garlic in the skillet for about 1 minute, or until fragrant.
6. Stir-fry the broccoli florets in the skillet for 3-4 minutes, or until they are bright green and tender-crisp.
7. Pour the sauce mixture over the cooked beef in the skillet. Stir everything together to evenly coat the steak and broccoli.
8. Cook for another 1-2 minutes, or until the sauce thickens.
9. Season to taste with salt and pepper.
10. Remove the lean beef stir-fry with broccoli and ginger from the heat and serve over cooked rice.

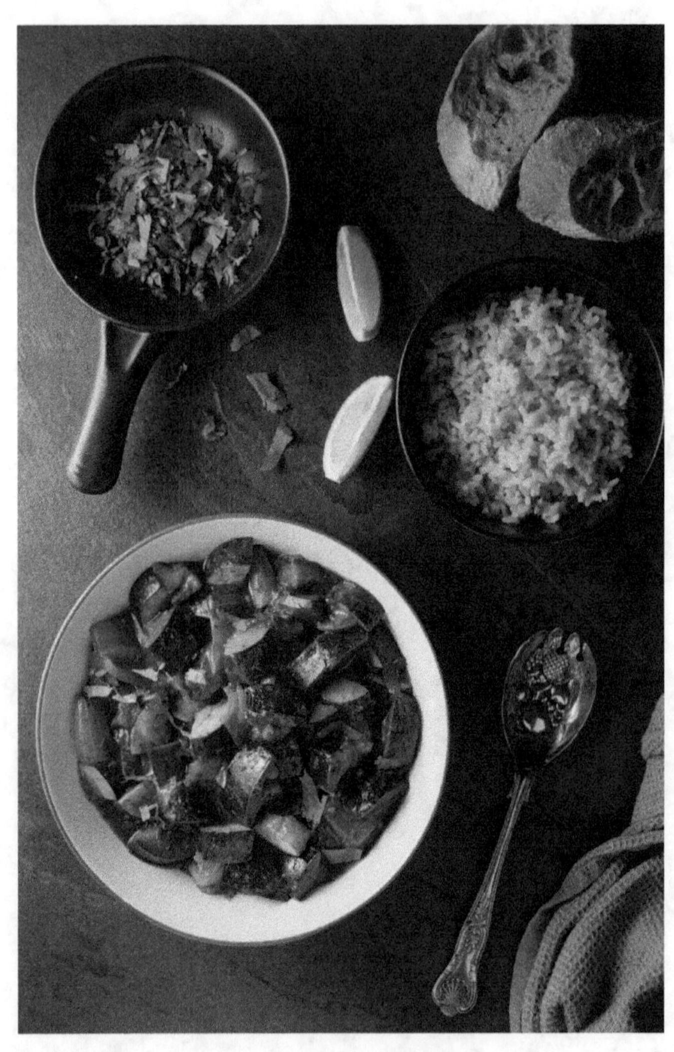

CHAPTER 7: BREAD AND GRAINS

Whole wheat bread

Ingredients:

- 3 cups whole wheat flour
- 1 cup all-purpose flour
- 2 1/4 teaspoons active dry yeast
- 2 tablespoons honey
- 2 tablespoons olive oil
- 1 1/2 teaspoons salt
- 1 3/4 cups warm water (110°F/43°C)

Instructions:

1. Combine the whole wheat flour, all-purpose flour, and salt in a large mixing basin.
2. Dissolve the yeast in warm water in a separate basin. Allow it to settle for 5 minutes or until foamy.
3. Stir in the honey and olive oil to the yeast mixture.

4. Combine the yeast and flour mixture in a mixing dish. Stir the dough until it comes together.

5. Transfer the dough to a floured board and knead for 8-10 minutes, or until smooth and elastic.

6. Cover the dough with a clean dish towel and place it in an oiled basin. Allow it to rise for about 1 hour in a warm environment, or until it doubles in size.

7. Preheat the oven to 375 degrees Fahrenheit (190 degrees Celsius).

8. To remove any air bubbles from the risen dough, punch it down. Turn the dough out onto a lightly floured board and form it into a loaf.

9. Place the formed dough in a loaf pan that has been oiled. Cover with a cloth and leave it to rise for another 30-45 minutes, or until it is slightly higher than the rim of the pan.

10. Bake the bread for 30-35 minutes, or until the top is golden brown and the loaf sounds hollow when tapped.

11. Remove the bread from the oven and set it aside to cool for a few minutes in the pan. After that, place it on a wire rack to cool entirely before slicing.

Brown rice

Ingredients:

- 1 cup brown rice
- 2 cups water
- 1/2 teaspoon salt (optional)

Instructions:

1. Rinse the brown rice by placing it in a fine-mesh strainer or colander and rinsing it under cold water until the water runs clear. This step aids in the removal of any debris or extra starch from the rice.
2. Soak the rice (optional): Soaking brown rice can improve its texture and shorten the cooking time. This step is optional, although it is suggested for the best results. Fill a bowl halfway with water and add the washed rice. Allow it to soak for 30 minutes before draining.
3. Cook the rice: Combine the soaked or rinsed rice, water, and salt (if needed) in a medium pot. Over medium-high heat, bring the mixture to a boil.
4. Reduce the heat to low and cover the pot with a tight-fitting lid after the water reaches a boil. Allow the rice to cook for 45-50 minutes, or until soft. Lifting the cover while the rice is cooking may cause

steam to escape and may result in uneven cooking.

5. Fluff the rice: When the rice is done, remove it from the fire and set it aside, covered, for 5 minutes. Remove the lid and gently fluff the rice with a fork. This process aids in the separation of the grains and the removal of any surplus moisture.

6. Brown rice is adaptable and can be served as a side dish or as a base for a variety of recipes. It goes well with vegetables, beans, stir-fried foods, curries, and any other main entrée of your choosing.

Quinoa

Ingredients:

- 1 cup quinoa
- 2 cups water
- 1 small red onion, thinly sliced
- 1 red bell pepper, diced
- 1 yellow bell pepper, diced
- 1 zucchini, sliced
- 1 cup cherry tomatoes, halved
- 2 tablespoons olive oil
- 1 tablespoon balsamic vinegar
- 1 tablespoon fresh lemon juice
- 2 tablespoons fresh parsley, chopped

- Salt and pepper to taste

Instructions:

1. Preheat the oven to 400 degrees Fahrenheit (200 degrees Celsius). On a baking sheet, arrange the sliced red onion, chopped red and yellow bell peppers, and sliced zucchini. Season with salt and pepper and drizzle with olive oil. Toss to evenly coat the vegetables.
2. Roast the vegetables for 20-25 minutes, or until soft and slightly caramelized, in a preheated oven. Set aside to cool after removing from the oven.
3. Rinse the quinoa in cold water to remove any bitterness while the vegetables cook. Combine the quinoa and water in a saucepan. Bring to a boil, then lower to a low heat, cover, and cook for 15 minutes, or until all of the water has been absorbed and the quinoa is soft. Remove from the heat and set aside to cool.
4. Combine the cooked quinoa and roasted vegetables in a large mixing basin. Combine the halved cherry tomatoes, fresh parsley, balsamic vinegar, and lemon juice in a mixing bowl. Gently toss to mix.

5. Season the quinoa salad to taste with salt and pepper. If desired, adjust the seasoning and add extra olive oil or lemon juice.
6. Allow the salad to sit for about 10-15 minutes to allow the flavors to blend. Chill or serve at room temperature.

Oatmeal

Ingredients:

- 1 cup rolled oats
- 2 cups water or milk (dairy or plant-based)
- Pinch of salt (optional)
- Sweeteners and toppings of your choice (e.g., honey, maple syrup, fresh fruits, nuts, seeds)

Instructions:

1. Bring the water or milk to a boil in a saucepan over medium heat.
2. To the boiling liquid, add the rolled oats and salt. Stir thoroughly.
3. Reduce the heat to low and continue to cook the oats for 5 minutes, stirring regularly. Simmer for a few minutes longer if you prefer a thicker consistency.

4. Remove the pot from the heat after the oatmeal has reached the appropriate consistency.
5. Sweeten your oats to taste with honey, maple syrup, or your favorite sweetener. Stir thoroughly.
6. Place the oatmeal in serving bowls.
7. Toppings such as fresh fruits, nuts, and seeds can be added to your oatmeal. Get creative and include everything you want!
8. Allow the oatmeal to cool for a few minutes before serving. It's scorching!

Barley

Ingredients:

- 1 cup barley
- 2 tablespoons olive oil
- 1 onion, chopped
- 2 carrots, diced
- 2 celery stalks, diced
- 3 cloves garlic, minced
- 6 cups vegetable or chicken broth
- 1 bay leaf
- 1 teaspoon dried thyme
- Salt and pepper to taste
- Fresh parsley, chopped (for garnish)

Instructions:

1. Rinse and drain the barley thoroughly in cold water.
2. Warm the olive oil in a big pot over medium heat. Mix in the chopped onion, carrots, and celery. Cook for 5 minutes, or until the vegetables soften.
3. Cook for an additional minute, or until the garlic is aromatic.
4. Pour in the rinsed barley and mix to incorporate with the vegetables.
5. Add the bay leaf and dried thyme to the vegetable or chicken broth. Season to taste with salt and pepper.
6. Bring the soup to a boil, then lower to a low heat. Cover the saucepan and cook for 45 minutes to an hour, or until the barley is cooked.
7. Remove the bay leaf from the saucepan after the barley is done. Season with salt and pepper to taste.
8. Garnish the barley soup with fresh parsley and serve immediately.

Buckwheat

Ingredients:

- 1 cup buckwheat groats

- 2 cups water
- 1/2 teaspoon salt
- 1 tablespoon butter or oil (optional)

Instructions:

1. To get rid of any dirt, rinse the buckwheat groats with cold water. Flow freely.
2. Bring the water to a boil in a medium-sized saucepan.
3. Boiling water is added along the salt and the rinsed buckwheat groats. Stir thoroughly.
4. Buckwheat should simmer for about 15-20 minutes, or until the groats are soft and have absorbed the majority of the water, on low heat with the lid on the pan. Depending on how soft or chewy you prefer your buckwheat, you can change the cooking time.
5. After the buckwheat has finished cooking, turn off the heat and let the pan remain, covered, for about five minutes to let the grains steam.
6. If desired, add a spoonful of butter or oil to the buckwheat to give it some richness.
7. Before serving, fluff the buckwheat with a fork.
8. It is possible to use buckwheat as a side dish or as a foundation for different toppings and seasonings. It can be used as

a base for salads, added to stir-fries, or enjoyed as a warm side dish with roasted veggies.

Savory Millet Pilaf

Ingredients:

- 1 cup millet
- 2 cups vegetable broth
- 1 tablespoon olive oil
- 1 small onion, finely chopped
- 2 cloves garlic, minced
- 1 carrot, diced
- 1 bell pepper, diced
- 1 zucchini, diced
- 1 teaspoon dried thyme
- 1 teaspoon ground cumin
- Salt and pepper to taste
- Fresh parsley, chopped (for garnish)

Instructions:

1. Drain the millet carefully after rinsing it in cold water.
2. The olive oil should be heated in a sizable pot over medium heat. When aromatic and transparent, add the minced onion and garlic.

3. The pot should now contain the diced zucchini, bell pepper, and carrot. The vegetables should be somewhat tender after a few minutes in the sauté pan.
4. Stir the millet with the oil and veggies in the pan after adding it.
5. Add the ground cumin and dried thyme after adding the vegetable broth. To taste, add salt and pepper to the food.
6. Heat should be turned down once the mixture comes to a boil. When the millet is cooked and has absorbed the liquid, simmer it for about 20 minutes with the cover on the pan.
7. To give the flavors time to blend, turn off the heat and let the pot remain, covered, for an additional five minutes.
8. With a fork, fluff the millet pilaf before transferring it to a serving bowl.
9. Before serving, garnish with freshly cut parsley.

Whole grain pasta

Ingredients:

- 8 ounces (225g) of whole grain pasta
- 2 tablespoons of olive oil

- 3 cloves of garlic, minced
- 1 small onion, finely chopped
- 1 bell pepper, thinly sliced
- 1 zucchini, thinly sliced
- 1 cup of cherry tomatoes, halved
- 1 cup of spinach leaves
- 1/4 teaspoon of red pepper flakes (optional)
- Salt and black pepper to taste
- Grated Parmesan cheese for serving (optional)

Instructions:

1. Large saucepan of salted water should be brought to a boil. As directed on the package, add the whole-wheat pasta and simmer until al dente. Drain, then set apart.
2. Olive oil should be heated in a sizable skillet over medium heat. Add the minced garlic and onion, and cook until aromatic and just beginning to turn golden.
3. Bell pepper and zucchini should be added to the skillet and cooked for 3–4 minutes, or until they begin to soften.
4. Add the spinach leaves and cherry tomatoes, stir, and simmer for an additional 2 to 3 minutes, or until the spinach wilts and the tomatoes start to soften.

5. For a little heat, if wanted, add the red pepper flakes. To taste, add salt and black pepper to the food.
6. Toss the cooked whole grain pasta with the remaining ingredients in the skillet to thoroughly incorporate and distribute the veggies.
7. Whole grain pasta should be taken off the pan and served hot. If preferred, top with some grated Parmesan cheese.

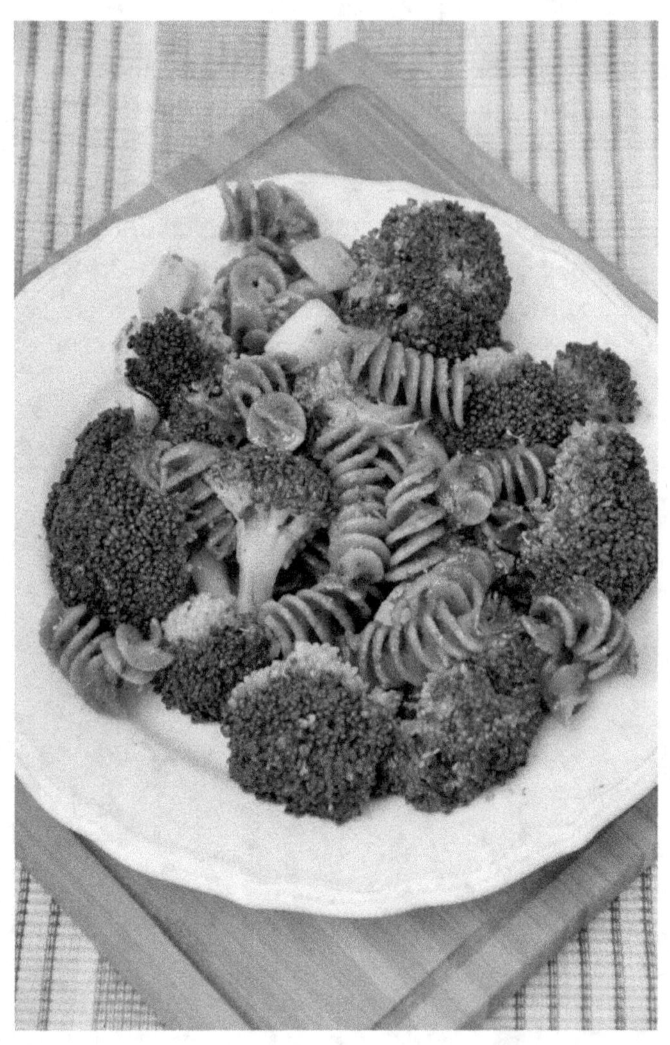

CHAPTER 8: DESSERTS AND TREATS

Ingredients:

2 cups of watermelon, cubed
2 cups of cantaloupe, cubed
2 cups of pineapple, cubed
2 cups of grapes, halved
2 cups of strawberries, sliced
2 cups of blueberries
2 cups of kiwi, peeled and sliced
1 tablespoon of fresh mint leaves, chopped (optional)
Juice of 1 lemon or lime (optional)

Instructions:

1. Under running water, thoroughly wash each fruit. Use paper towels or a clean kitchen towel to pat them dry.
2. Cut the watermelon, cantaloupe, and pineapple into bite-sized cubes after removing the rinds and seeds. Put them in a sizable bowl for mixing.

3. To the bowl of cubed fruits, add the grapes, strawberries, blueberries, and kiwi.
4. If you want to give the fruit salad a little tang, squeeze some lemon or lime juice over it. Gently stir the fruits to coat them.
5. If you're using fresh mint, finely chop some leaves and add them to the fruit salad. If you don't like mint, it is optional but offers a cool flavor.
6. Toss the fruit salad gently to properly distribute all the ingredients.
7. To allow the flavors to merge and the fruits to chill, cover the bowl with plastic wrap or move it to an airtight container and place it in the refrigerator for at least an hour.
8. To redistribute the liquids, gently mix the fruit salad once more right before serving.
9. In individual bowls or glasses, serve the fresh fruit salad and enjoy!

Yogurt parfait with berries and granola

Ingredients:

- 1 cup Greek yogurt
- 1 cup mixed berries (strawberries, blueberries, raspberries)
- 1/2 cup granola

- 2 tablespoons honey (optional)
- Fresh mint leaves for garnish (optional)

Instructions:

1. The berries should first be carefully cleaned. If desired, slice the strawberries and leave aside.
2. The parfait should be layered in a glass or dish. Greek yogurt should be the foundation at first.
3. To the yogurt, add a layer of mixed berries. With each variety of berry, you can make a layer or combine them.
4. Granola should be scattered on top of the berries. This gives the parfait a crunchy texture.
5. Until you have used up all the ingredients or have reached the desired height for the parfait, keep layering the yogurt, berries, and granola.
6. Pour some honey over each layer of the parfait if you'd like it to be sweeter. This step is not necessary because the berries already have a built-in sweetness.
7. Top off the parfait with one last granola sprinkle to complete it.
8. To add freshness and improve the look, you might garnish with a few fresh mint leaves.

9. Enjoy your healthy and energizing yogurt parfait with berries and granola right away!

cinnamon- and honey-infused baked apples

Ingredients:

- 4 medium-sized apples (preferably Granny Smith or Honeycrisp)
- 2 tablespoons unsalted butter, melted
- 2 tablespoons brown sugar
- 1 teaspoon ground cinnamon
- 1/4 teaspoon ground nutmeg
- 1/4 cup chopped nuts (such as walnuts or pecans)
- Honey for drizzling

Instructions:

1. Set your oven's temperature to 375°F (190°C). A baking dish should be lightly greased or lined with parchment paper.
2. After washing, pat the apples dry. Each apple is cored, the seeds are removed, and a hollow is created in the center to hold the filling. You can use a small paring knife or an apple corer.

3. Melted butter, brown sugar, cinnamon, and nutmeg should all be thoroughly mixed in a small basin.

4. The apples should be covered evenly with the melted butter mixture. Put the cored apples in the baking dish that has been prepared.

5. The chopped nuts should be placed in the apple's center cavity, gently pressed in.

6. Any leftover butter mixture should be sprinkled on top of the apples in the baking dish.

7. The dish should bake for about 25 to 30 minutes, or until the apples are soft and the filling is browned, in a preheated oven. By sticking a fork into the apples, you can determine when they are done; they should be soft but not mushy.

8. After removing the baked apples from the oven, give them some time to cool.

9. Warm the apples after baking. Just before serving, drizzle each apple with honey and, at your discretion, top with a little additional cinnamon for taste.

10. Enjoy your cinnamon- and honey-infused baked apples while they're still warm and comforting!

Chia seed pudding with almond milk and fruit topping

Ingredients:

- 1/4 cup chia seeds
- 1 cup almond milk (unsweetened)
- 1 tablespoon honey or maple syrup (optional, for sweetness)
- 1/2 teaspoon vanilla extract
- Assorted fresh fruits (such as berries, sliced bananas, mango, or peaches)
- Nuts or shredded coconut for garnish (optional)

Instructions:

1. Chia seeds, almond milk, honey or maple syrup (if used), and vanilla extract should all be combined in a medium basin. To make sure the chia seeds are dispersed equally, stir thoroughly. Give the mixture five minutes to rest.
2. To avoid clumping, stir the chia seed mixture once more after 5 minutes. Place the bowl in the fridge for at least two hours or overnight. Cover it. In this way, the liquid can be absorbed by the chia seeds, which then thicken into a pudding-like consistency.

3. Give the chia seed pudding a thorough stir after it has dried to remove any clumps. You can add a bit extra almond milk to the pudding to thin it down if it is too thick for your tastes.
4. Put the chia seed pudding into dishes or glasses for serving. Add your favorite fresh fruits, like berries, banana slices, mango, or peaches, on top. For additional texture and flavor, add some nuts or coconut shreds.
5. Chia seed pudding can be served right away or put back in the fridge to wait to be served. You can eat the pudding either cold or at room temperature.

Dark chocolate-covered strawberries

Ingredients:

- 1 pound of fresh strawberries
- 8 ounces of dark chocolate (70% cocoa or higher)
- Optional toppings: chopped nuts, shredded coconut, sprinkles, etc.

Instructions:

1. The strawberries should be cleaned and dried with paper towels. Before dipping

them in chocolate, make certain they are totally dry.

2. Use wax paper or parchment paper to cover a baking sheet.

3. Put the broken chunks of dark chocolate in a bowl that may be heated in the microwave. Stirring in between, microwave in 30-second intervals until the chocolate is totally melted and smooth. As an alternative, you might use a double boiler over a cooktop to melt the chocolate.

4. Each strawberry should be held by the stem or dipped into the molten chocolate using a toothpick, then completely coated. Let any extra chocolate fall off.

5. Put the strawberry covered in chocolate on the baking sheet that has been prepared. The remaining strawberries should be used in a similar manner.

6. Before the chocolate hardens, if desired, top the chocolate-covered strawberries with your preferred garnishes.

7. Place the baking sheet in the refrigerator for about 30 minutes, or until the chocolate has firm, after coating all the strawberries.

8. The strawberries can be taken out of the fridge and served right away once the chocolate has set. If you won't be serving them right away, you can keep them in

the fridge for up to two days in an airtight container.

Frozen banana bites

Ingredients:

- 3 ripe bananas
- 1/2 cup dark chocolate chips or chopped dark chocolate
- 1/4 cup unsweetened shredded coconut (optional)
- 1/4 cup chopped nuts (such as almonds, peanuts, or walnuts) (optional)
- Wooden skewers or toothpicks

Instructions:

1. Bananas should be peeled and chopped into bite-sized pieces. Each banana chunk should have a wooden skewer or toothpick in it. They should be frozen for approximately an hour, or until they are solid, on a baking sheet coated with parchment paper.
2. Melt the dark chocolate chips or chopped dark chocolate in a bowl that can go in the microwave. To make this, microwave the chocolate in 30-second intervals while

stirring, until it is totally melted and smooth.

3. Spread out chopped or shredded nuts or coconut on a small plate or shallow dish if using.
4. Each piece of frozen banana should be dipped into the melted chocolate and well covered. All extra chocolate should drip off.
5. If preferred, roll the chocolate-coated banana chunk in shredded coconut or finely chopped almonds right away, gently pressing the coating to help the nuts stick. The remaining banana pieces should be used in a similar manner.
6. Back on the parchment-lined baking sheet, reposition the frozen covered banana bits. At least two hours or until they are completely frozen, freeze.
7. Transfer the frozen banana bites to an airtight container or a freezer bag that can be sealed for storage.
8. As a cool and tasty treat, serve the frozen banana bites straight from the freezer.

Greek yogurt popsicles with fruit puree

Ingredients:

- 2 cups Greek yogurt

- 1/4 cup honey or maple syrup (adjust to taste)
- 1 teaspoon vanilla extract
- 1 cup fruit of your choice (e.g., strawberries, blueberries, mango, etc.)
- 1 tablespoon lemon juice (optional)

Instructions:

1. The fruit of your choice should be pureed until smooth in a blender or food processor. If necessary, you can add a tablespoon of lemon juice to improve the flavor and stop fruits like apples or bananas from turning brown.
2. Greek yogurt, honey (or maple syrup), and vanilla extract should all be combined in a mixing basin. Well combine till creamy and smooth.
3. Fill the Greek yogurt mixture halfway into your popsicle molds.
4. Fill each mold to the brim with the fruit puree before spooning it on top of the yogurt mixture. To create a marbled appearance, stir the yogurt and fruit together with a popsicle stick or toothpick.
5. Make sure the popsicle sticks are centered and standing properly when you insert them into each mold.

6. Place the molds in the freezer, and allow them to stay there until completely solid, at least 4-6 hours.
7. After the popsicles have frozen, you can remove them from the molds by immersing them quickly in warm water or running warm water over the bottom of the molds. Take the popsicles out of the molds slowly.
8. Serve right away or freeze the popsicles in plastic bags or an airtight container for later consumption.

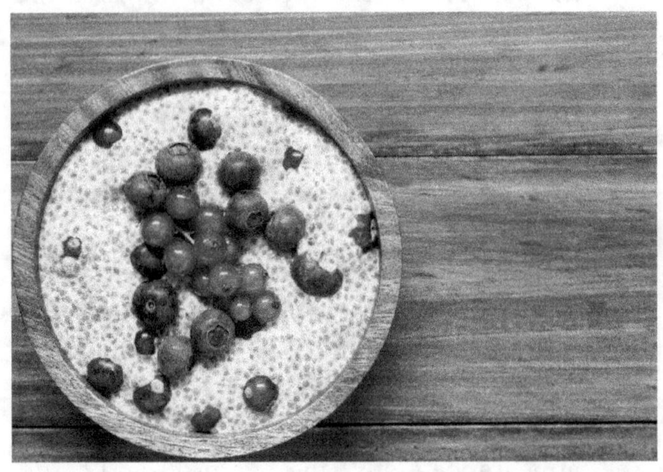

Conclusion

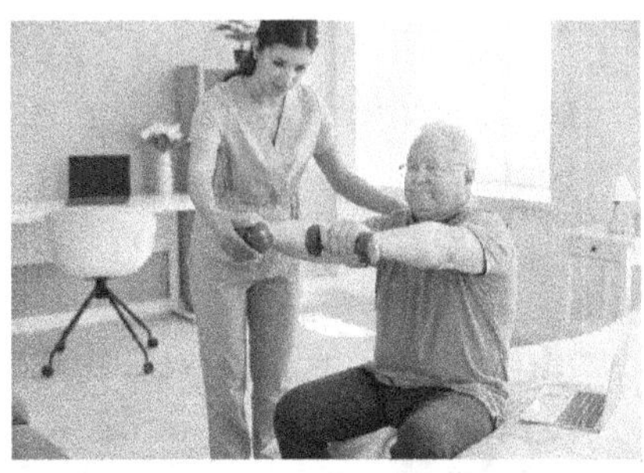

Although managing arthritis can be difficult, there are many tools at people's disposal to help them manage their illness and enhance their quality of life. Along with medical interventions, there are a number of educational resources, support networks, and online forums that provide helpful knowledge, advice, and emotional support. These extra resources can be really beneficial whether you're looking for guidance on how to manage symptoms, investigating alternative therapies, or searching for a supportive community. Here are some alternatives to think about:

The Arthritis Foundation is a well-known foundation that offers comprehensive resources for persons with arthritis. Their website provides access to nearby support groups as well as educational articles, workout plans, and self-management advice. In order to encourage research and raise awareness about arthritis, they also plan events and advocacy campaigns.

The NIAMS, or National Institute of Arthritis and Musculoskeletal and Skin Diseases The National Institutes of Health (NIH) division known as NIAMS is dedicated to studying, preventing, and treating musculoskeletal disorders like arthritis. Their website provides comprehensive details on different types of arthritis, available treatments, ongoing clinical trials, and resources for medical professionals.

Online Support Communities: Getting involved in arthritis-specific forums and support groups online can give you a sense of belonging and a way to meet people going through comparable struggles. Forums are available on websites like Arthritis-Health, CreakyJoints, and Inspire where people may share their stories, ask questions, and get support from other arthritis sufferers.

Exercise regimens and physical treatment: Physical therapy is essential for treating arthritic symptoms. To create a customized workout plan that emphasizes flexibility, strength, and joint protection, speak with a physical therapist who specializes in arthritis. In addition, the Arthritis Foundation provides sessions that include water-based exercises like swimming or aquatic fitness for adults with arthritis.

Complementary and Alternative Medicine (CAM): As a complement to conventional medicines, many people with arthritis look into complementary and alternative therapies. Evidence-based information on the safety and effectiveness of various CAM strategies, such as acupuncture, herbal medicines, and mind-body exercises like yoga and meditation, is available from resources like the National Center for Complementary and Integrative Health (NCCIH).

Occupational therapy can help people with arthritis modify their circumstances to lessen joint stress and enhance daily functioning. They offer energy-saving tips, ergonomic advice, and assistive technology to make chores simpler. To locate licensed occupational therapists in your region, use the resources provided by the American Occupational Therapy Association (AOTA).

Mobile applications for tracking symptoms, medications, and physical activity are available for people with arthritis. Additionally, some apps offer instructional materials, pain treatment methods, and fitness videos. MyRA,

ArthritisPower, and Arthritis App are a few examples.

publications and Publications: There are a lot of publications that provide insights into life with arthritis as well as useful tips. Grant Cooper's "The Arthritis Handbook: Improve Your Health and Manage the Pain of Osteoarthritis" and Tammi L. Shlotzhauer's "Living with Rheumatoid Arthritis" are two well-known works. These websites might offer practical advice and coping mechanisms for managing arthritis on a daily basis.

Never try a new treatment or make any significant modifications to your arthritis management strategy without first consulting your healthcare professional. These other resources can be helpful additions to your medical treatment, offering guidance, encouragement, and support while you manage your arthritis.

www.ingramcontent.com/pod-product-compliance
Lightning Source LLC
Chambersburg PA
CBHW070847260726
48661CB00004B/1293